Elderly Care

Towards Holistic Nursing

USING NURSING MODELS SERIES

General Editors:

Susan E Norman SRN, DNCert, RNT
Senior Tutor, The Nightingale School, St Thomas's Hospital, London
Computer Assisted Learning (CAL) Project Leader

Jane E Schober SRN, RCNT, DipN Ed, DipN (Lond), RNT
Tutor, Nursing Studies, Institute of Advanced Nursing Education, Royal
College of Nursing

Christine Webb BA, MSc, PhD, SRN, RSCN, RNT
Principal Lecturer in Nursing, Department of Nursing, Health and Applied
Social Studies, Bristol Polytechnic, Bristol

The views expressed in this book are those of the authors of individual chapters
and do not necessarily reflect the opinions of the series editors.

Elderly Care
Towards Holistic Nursing

Jane Easterbrook
MA, RGN, STD, RCNT, DipEd

Assistant Director of Nurse Education,
Head of Staff Development, The Nightingale
School, St. Thomas's Hospital,
London

HODDER AND STOUGHTON
LONDON SYDNEY AUCKLAND TORONTO

Elderly care.—(Using nursing models
  series).
  1. Geriatric nursing
  I. Easterbrook, Jane   II. Series
  610.73'65   RC954

  ISBN 0 340 38036 5

First published 1987

Typeset by Macmillan India Ltd., Bangalore 560 025

Printed in Great Britain
for Hodder and Stoughton Educational,
a division of Hodder and Stoughton Ltd,
Mill Road, Dunton Green, Sevenoaks, Kent TN13 2YD
by Page Bros (Norwich) Ltd

Table of Contents

List of Contributors

Mrs Jane Chapman obtained a degree in Social Science and Administration at the University of London in 1977, and completed her nurse training at the Middlesex Hospital in 1979. In 1980 she went to the Nursing Practice Research Unit as a Research Assistant on a DHSS funded project surveying the current treatments of established pressure sores. During this time Mrs Chapman also conducted a piece of research aimed at developing methods for the assessment of nutritional status of elderly patients. In 1983 Mrs Chapman became a mother, but retained links with nursing research through lecturing, and teaching Unit 5 for the Diploma in Nursing Studies at the Royal College of Nursing. Since 1985 she has been Research Nurse for the Computer Assisted Learning Project at the Nightingale School, St Thomas' Hospital.

Miss Ann Bergen obtained her first degree in History at the University of Reading in 1974. She completed her nurse training at Addenbrooke's Hospital in Cambridge in 1978. From 1979 until 1984 she worked with the elderly as a Staff Nurse, and then as a Sister, on an acute assessment ward at Northwick Park Hospital, Harrow, during which time she studied for the Diploma in Nursing (new curriculum) at the Royal College of Nursing. In 1984 Miss Bergen undertook District Nurse training at the West London Institute of Higher Education and is currently practising as a District Nursing Sister with Harrow Health Authority.

Dr Alan Pearson has had a wealth of experience both in the United Kingdom and abroad. Following completion of his Master of Science Degree at the University of Manchester, he took up the post of Senior Nurse, Clinical Practice Development, Burford Community Hospital and Nursing Development Unit. The innovative nursing work in this area is well known. Dr Pearson was awarded his PhD by the University of London in 1985, and was also elected as a Fellow of the Royal College of Nursing. He has just been appointed Professor of Nursing and Foundation Dean, Faculty of Nursing, Deakin University, Geelong, Victoria, Australia.

Mr Alan Skeath has had a varied career in psychiatric nursing, both in this country and abroad. He has been a Nurse Tutor for many years, and his experience includes being an examiner to the General Nursing Council. He was awarded a Masters Degree in Education by the University of London in 1981 and is currently Director of Nurse Education at Dewsbury School of Nursing.

Mrs Mary Watkins completed her general nurse training in 1976 at Westminster Hospital, and subsequently undertook mental nurse training at the Maudsley Hospital in 1977. Mrs Watkins has had experience as a teacher, both at the basic and post-basic level and is currently working as a tutor (In-service Education and Training), at the Maudsley Hospital School of Nursing. She completed the Diploma in Nursing (new curriculum) in 1985 and is currently undertaking the Masters Degree in Nursing at the University of Wales. Mrs Watkins was successful in achieving a Florence Nightingale Memorial Scholarship this year, to examine nursing models and psychiatric curricula in Britain and the USA. In May 1987, Mrs Watkins will be taking up a joint appointment with the Institute of Advanced Nursing Education and the Nightingale School of Nursing.

Miss Alison Binnie completed her nurse training in 1975 and has had widespread nursing experience in various nursing specialties. From 1981 until 1984 Miss Binnie was the Nursing Process Co-ordinator with the Cambridge Health District. Since 1984 she has been the Senior Sister on a Surgical Unit at the John Radcliffe Hospital in Oxford where she is not only responsible for the running of her own ward, but also for developing nursing practice in a unit of three wards. Miss Binnie completed the Diploma in Nursing (new curriculum) at the Royal College of Nursing in 1985. Her special interest at present is planning the development of primary nursing in the acute surgical setting.

Dr Ann Faulkner is well known as a writer and teacher. Her research work in the area of communication is of particular note, and she is currently Director of the Communication in Nursing Education Project. Her special interest is improving nurses' skills when communicating with people who have cancer. Dr Faulkner is currently working as a Senior Lecturer in the Department of Nursing Studies at the University of Edinburgh.

Acknowledgements

The editor would like to thank the following for permission to reproduce material:

Churchill Livingstone
Controller of Her Majesty's Stationery Office
Pergamon Press

Foreword

There have been a large number of social and economic changes in the United Kingdom during the past twenty five years. Two particular changes have had a direct impact on elderly care; an increase in the number of married women who work, and an increased number of elderly people who themselves live longer.

In many instances the network of family support mechanisms, which once surrounded the elderly person, no longer exists. It might be argued that it is more appropriate for such specialist care to be provided by those properly prepared, and that the role of friends/relatives should rightfully be to augment the work of qualified staff.

It is interesting that, unlike any other client group at this time, the elderly are grouped together, regardless of their state of health, or nature of disease. This approach has advantages. Interlinks between the many facets are more easily made by persons who, of necessity, require a wide preparation. It also has disadvantages. Particular sets of signs, symptoms and circumstances become linked with a particular age group when in fact, these may occur from adulthood onwards. Indeed, the needs of elderly persons have great similarity with the needs of other adults, but the methods of meeting such needs may require modification. However, it is quite inappropriate to attempt to identify such modifications by age group alone.

Many occupational groups contribute to elderly care; nursing is one of them. As is specifically identified in Chapter 6, unless appropriate procedures are used to co-ordinate the various activities, the resulting care is less than effective. All nursing care encompasses several types of activity: prevention of disease; undertaking activities when a person is prevented by illness from carrying out these personally; taking specific actions which are necessary because of the type of illness; and assisting the individual to return to the degree of independence possible.

Although the elderly are described as a group, it must be remembered that each member of the group has a unique identity. To be able to provide meaningful care, it is essential to consider the totality of each person, as an individual, within his/her immediate circle of friends/family, and within the wider groups in society. In Chapter 1, the holistic approach to care is re-emphasised and demonstrated.

Nursing elderly persons is, therefore, a complex matter. Some 'tools' exist to assist the nurse in his/her provision of care; nursing models are one important group of 'tools' but these remain under-used: Perhaps this is not surprising. The seemingly complicated nature of the models may make it difficult for nurses to transfer knowledge of them into practice. This book's contributors have recognised such difficulties and have attempted to overcome them by providing clear explanations, linked with examples, of their application to individual care. Some of these examples show the provision of excellent care; others discuss difficulties in elderly care provision and how, to some extent, they may be overcome by a logical, structured approach to care.

The very nature of the practical applications used raises the question of why it is possible for some to follow this route, even in the face of many difficulties, whilst many do not. Some nurses have argued the impossibility of such approaches, given the manpower problems. But if these helpful tools are not being used to inform and guide practice, is the most effective use of time and resources being made?

With the increasing number of elderly persons in the population, all nurses will be involved in some aspect of their care. Every registered nurse is professionally accountable for providing the highest standards of care. To this end, this book will be welcomed by all nurses who strive to meet this goal in their work with elderly persons.

J Peta Allan
DipFEd, MA, RGN, ONC, RNT, FBIM

Introduction

To say that this is a book solely about nursing models would be to stray from the truth. This volume is dedicated to the older person. Nursing models are secondary to this central process, and are considered only in the light in which they may inform, guide and develop nursing practice. In a sense, this book should hold appeal for nurses working within most specialties since, with the exception of maternity and child care, all nurses have contact with individuals who are in the later stages of their lives.

This contact is likely to escalate, as there is little doubt that the world is growing older. This is not because older people are in general living longer, but is due to the improvement in the quality of life that people can expect in their early years. It is the resultant reduction in infant mortality that is largely responsible for the increasing numbers of children who can expect to live a full lifespan. Just to illustrate this last point, at the turn of the century, a male child at birth could expect to live marginally over 48 years. A female child did slightly better at 52 years. However, during the 1970s, this life expectancy increased to 70 and 76 years respectively (Central Statistical Office, 1977).

It has also been pointed out by Abrams (1978) that the number of very elderly people in our society will increase dramatically over the next few decades. Thus, the reader may identify a more personal interest, since many of us are likely to be within that group. Whether this will be a happy or miserable experience during a period of illness will depend on how the art and science of nursing are analysed, criticised and directed today.

However, it is readily acknowledged that it is no easy task to face the prospect of advancing years and death, and the situation is not helped by a society which urges both men and women to look as young as possible for as long as possible. A negative attitude towards ageing may be one of the reasons for the lack of initiative on the part of nursing to recognise elderly care as a specialist branch of that discipline.

As long ago as 1946, Doctor Marjorie Warren recommended geriatrics as a specialty comparable with paediatrics. This need was echoed by the Royal College of Nursing (1975) and the World Health Organization (1976). However, although it was a compulsory experience for their pupil nurse colleagues, elderly care was not included in the syllabus for student nurses until 1973. Even then, this particular unit of learning remained optional. It was not until 1977 that the inclusion of a module specifically designed to initiate all basic learners in this area of care became a reality.

The emergence of specific post basic education for professional nurses directly concerned with care of the elderly has been even more haphazard. Only after the Joint Board of Clinical Nursing Studies was established in 1970 were course centres required to demonstrate quality in both the clinical experience offered and the taught component, in order to receive validation from the Board and thus run nationally recognized courses. More recent developments adding to the body of nursing knowledge include the excellent material produced by the Open University in the course 'An Ageing Population', and the Diploma in Gerontology held under the auspices of the University of London.

During the 1970s then, there was a recognition of the elderly as a group with special needs. Now, through the values reflected in conceptual frameworks for a nursing process approach to care, a further step forward has been made. At last, there is a growing acceptance of the older person as an individual with a unique biography which needs to be taken into account in both the prevention of, and care during, periods of ill health. The development of nursing models is important in this process, since they provide the profession with a theoretical basis for education, management, practice and research. It is not intended here to categorise the bewildering array of models that face nurses studying at an advanced level. Webb (1986) gives an excellent presentation which would be difficult to match.

It is pointed out here, however, that theory development is not new. Nurses often have personalised views of some particular aspect of nursing care. Indeed, McFarlane (1977) comments that if nurses were to write down the information they have gathered in years of experience, nursing would possess a wealth of knowledge. However, this informal and often unrecorded theory may seem to be of limited use. If theory is to be used to explain, predict and control nursing, then it must be testable by others, eventually adding to the body of nursing knowledge.

This then is what the contributors to this book offer. The aim is not only to stimulate thought and discussion, but also to offer the opportunity for professional nurses to analyse nursing situations where the care of the older person is involved. To do this with any measure of meaning, an analytical framework is essential. In other words, at least to begin with, it is helpful to know what questions to ask of any model. To augment this process Aggleton and Chalmers (1984) provide an excellent beginning.

The use of nursing models presents opportunities for nurses to deliver care for individuals in a unique and creative way. If the reader is looking for a perfect example, yet another mechanistic stereotype for the delivery of care, then disappointment is likely. It is fully accepted that differences in opinion about the way in which each author has used the model will be expressed. This is healthy, since it is only through this kind of debate that professional growth can be realized.

My gratitude is extended to the authors for the enormous amount of hard work that each chapter demonstrates. My grateful thanks are also due to the series editors for their counsel, patience and good humour.

JE, 1987

References

Abrams M 1978 *Beyond three score and ten: a first report on a survey of the elderly.* Age Concern, Mitcham.

Aggleton P & Chalmers H 1984 Models and theories: defining the terms. *Nursing Times*, **80**, 36: 24–28.

Central Statistical Office 1977 *Social trends no. 8.* HMSO, London.

McFarlane J 1977 Developing a theory of nursing: the relation of theory to practice, evaluation and research. *Journal of Advanced Nursing*, **2**: 261–271.

Royal College of Nursing 1975 *Improving geriatric care in hospitals.* RCN, London.

Warren M 1946 Care of the chronic aged sick. *The Lancet*, June 8th: 841–843.

Webb C 1986 *Women's Health.* Hodder & Stoughton, Sevenoaks.

World Health Organization 1976 *Summary of a report of a working group on nursing aspects in care of the elderly.* WHO, Geneva.

I

A problem of nutrition: an extension of Roper's Activities of Living model

Jane Chapman

There is considerable research evidence available to indicate that the nutritional care of hospitalised elderly patients does not receive all the attention that it should. In fact the findings suggest that many elderly patients receive much less than the recommended daily intake (RDI) of calories and nutrients while in hospital, thus putting them at risk of developing either frank, or at least sub-clinical malnutrition during a hospital stay. Sub-clinical malnutrition is defined as a sub-optimal level of blood constituents, demonstrated biochemically, or a sub-optimal level of nutrient intake as compared with the recommended daily intake (DHSS 1969). With the current drive to keep the elderly out of hospital (and other caring institutions) and in the community, the desirability of discharging patients in a well nourished state, with the skills and knowledge necessary to maintain an adequate intake, is only too obvious.

Background and research

It is readily accepted that there is some argument amongst the 'experts' as to what the recommended intake of calories and nutrients for an elderly person should be, so for the sake of consistency the guidelines used in this chapter are those suggested by the DHSS (1969). These levels have been derived from the recommended intake levels for younger adults with an allowance made for the average rate of decline associated with advancing age (Table 1.1). When looking at the intake figures for hospitalised patients it must be remembered that although activity may be reduced due to the confines of the ward, intake

Table 1.1 Recommended daily intake of energy nutrients for elderly people in the UK (DHSS 1969)

	Men		Women	
	65–74 years	75+ years	65–74 years	75+ years
Energy (kcal)	2350	2100	2050	1900
Protein (g)	59	53	51	48
Calcium (mg)	500	500	500	500
Iron (mg)	10	10	10	10
Vitamin C (mg)	30	30	30	30

requirements may in fact be higher than the accepted average if the patient is recovering from any form of illness, infection, trauma or surgery. Since Cuthbertson (1932) first identified the catabolic effect of trauma, it has been recognised that a level of protein and calorie intake well above the RDI is required post trauma.

Findings of British studies

A comprehensive review of the literature from 1975 to 1984 using the MEDLINE automated literature search facility revealed a total of 23 British studies which reported intake levels below the DHSS recommendation amongst samples of hospitalised elderly patients. Three studies have been selected to illustrate the research in this field.

Evans and Stock (1971) examined individually weighed total food intakes over a period of 8 days for a sample of 19 men and 25 women (age range 61–94 years). They divided their sample into three groups according to the nursing/medical care objective:

Group 1 long stay (continuing care)
Group 2 acutely ill/short stay
Group 3 rehabilitation/ready for discharge

They found that the mean energy intake was lower than the recommended daily intake for all three groups (RDI 2100 kcal, sample mean 1405 kcal). They also found that intakes of both calories and nutrients were significantly lower in Group 3, the self caring and generally the most active group, than for the patients in Groups 1 and 2. Possible reasons suggested for this are that the patients in this group make a poor choice of food, find the effort required to feed themselves restrictive, and insufficient time is allowed for eating. The highest intakes were recorded for patients in Group 1, who were generally the most dependent and required the most nursing attention. These issues will be discussed again later in the chapter.

The second study selected is the work of Older, Edwards and Dickerson (1980). They studied the voluntary nutrient intake of a sample of acutely ill women (age range 54–88 years, mean 78 years). All the patients were recovering from a surgical operation for the repair of a femoral neck fracture. Total nutrient intake was measured on days 3, 7 and 14 after the operation. They found that the mean intakes of protein, energy, Vitamin D, riboflavin, Vitamin C, thiamine and niacin fell short of the DHSS recommended levels. For example, on the seventh post-operative day, the mean energy intake was 1040 kcal, range 123–2275 kcal and mean protein intake 36.5 g, range 3.0–69.8 g (DHSS recommendations for 75+ years are 1900 kcal energy, 48 g protein).

Vir and Love (1979) conducted a survey of the voluntary food intake of 97 continuing care elderly inpatients in Northern Ireland for a period of 7 days. Their research findings are similar to those described above. Half the group received a vitamin supplement for three months prior to the survey and the others did not. Analysis of the data revealed that 17 per cent of

the supplemented group and 21 per cent of the non-supplemented group were consuming less than two-thirds of the RDI in terms of energy (calories), and that 64 per cent of the supplemented group and 91 per cent of the non-supplemented group were found biochemically to have some nutrient deficiency, that is, they had sub-clinical malnutrition. This situation is not necessarily a threat on its own, providing the person's equilibrium is stable; however, in the event of a life crisis such as an infection, accident or bereavement, sub-clinical malnutrition could swing the balance away from recovery and towards chronic disability, as the individual may not have the resources to combat the crisis.

The role of the nurse

Many nursing and medical textbooks agree that the nurse is the person largely responsible for the nutritional care of the individual patient (see, for example, Pearce 1975, Beck 1977, Davidson 1975). In hospital the patient is removed from the source of food and the nurse has to act as liaison between the patient and the catering services, by requesting appropriate foods for each patient, or by checking and sanctioning the patient's own choice of food. There is little evidence to imply that there is an actual nutritional shortfall in the food on offer in hospitals. Catering departments are vigorously controlled to supply food adequate both in quantity and quality to satisfy the needs of patients. The nurse is then in the best position to supervise the distribution of the meals and monitor the patients' intake. The research findings discussed above indicate that, for some elderly patients, the amount of food that they eat is not adequate to meet their needs (i.e. an intake level below the recommended level) and this suggests that the nurse is the weak link in the chain of nutritional care.

The author's own research (Chapman 1983) points to the fact that nutritional care is not seen as a priority by nursing staff. During a project to design a method for the assessment of mechanical problems associated with eating and drinking, a series of non-participant observation sessions were carried out on wards at lunchtime. Twenty-four elderly patients were studied (age range 68–90 years), four each from three geriatric, one orthopaedic, and two general medical wards. Each patient was observed on a maximum of six occasions. During data collection the activities of all the nursing staff on duty during each meal-time were also recorded. A total of 129 nurses were on duty during the 31 observation periods. A breakdown of the nurses' activities during the mealtime revealed that 40 per cent of the activities were not related to the meal at all (for example, bed making, Kardex writing, off ward throughout mealtime), 25 per cent of the activities included a check that each patient had a meal, but the remainder of the time was spent in other pursuits: only in 25 per cent of cases did the nursing staff monitor the mealtime and offer assistance where necessary. On the remaining 10 per cent of occasions, the nurses either talked amongst themselves and/or handed out menu cards for the next day, thus staying on the ward during the mealtime but taking no active part in the meal at all.

Older, Edwards and Dickerson (1980) report similar findings, stating that the nurses' evaluation of food intake was poor; a more serious threat to the patient was that there seemed to be no effective attempt by the nursing staff to improve patients' food intake, especially in those who consistently rejected food. The authors pointed out that although the elderly patient may have a fickle appetite, they usually respond to encouragement and assistance. (This is borne out by the study of care which follows.)

If the findings described above are representative of the situation for many elderly patients, then possible reasons for the threat to adequate nutrition are only too evident. Many nursing textbooks do indeed point to the nurse as the person responsible for the patients' nutritional care, but generally a passing reference to this situation is all that is made, e.g. Hector (1980) and Toohey (1981). What seems to be lacking is an adequate model for the provision of nutritional care for the elderly, a gap that this chapter seeks to fill.

Choosing an appropriate model

Nutritional care encompasses two main aims: firstly to ensure that patients receive adequate nourishment for their needs on a daily basis throughout the hospital stay, and secondly to provide the patient with the necessary skills and knowledge so that he may adequately provide himself with a balanced diet once released from hospital. This second aspect is particularly important when considering the care of the elderly, and sadly it is often overlooked. For example, in the author's own experience, nurses find themselves routinely cutting up food for a patient who has some problems performing this task, rather than trying to encourage the patient to master the skill (a rather longer process). To the medical staff, the patient may seem fit for discharge but may well have to return to hospital at a later date with another problem which can be directly related to a poor nutritional intake following discharge. Poor nutritional intake can lead to a variety of problems, for example lowered resistance to infection, so this link which could lead to the situation being repeated may not be directly apparent.

Adequate nutritional care requires accurate assessment of physical factors (relating to nutritional status), functional factors (relating to the ability to prepare and eat food) and social factors (relating to dietary habit, motivation to eat, enjoyment of eating and so on). Care planning should use this information to tailor the care to meet the individual's needs. It should be followed up by a regular programme of evaluation and review so that once problems have been identified, effort can be channelled into overcoming them and any new problem can be quickly identified and care altered accordingly.

For most elderly patients, nutrition is only one area of care with which nursing staff need to concern themselves. When at home, it is customary for people to fit the activities associated with eating and drinking into their pattern for daily living, rather than treating the activity as something 'special'. Therefore the choice of model has been made to encompass the following criteria:

1   It should allow care planning to take account of the individual's actual functional capabilities.
2   It should allow the individual's normal living pattern to be considered; eating and drinking do not take place in isolation from other activities (for example food preparation, socialising and communicating).
3   It should allow forward planning towards discharge/long term care to incorporate guidance towards sound nutritional practices which reflect the individual's future prospects.

The Roper model of nursing (1980) is based on functional assessment of the activities of living, together with a framework for interpretation of the assessment findings, planning and implementation of care, and evaluation of the effects of the care (the nursing process). This then, provides a good starting point for devising a model for nutritional care, as it specifically allows the nurse to plan with the patient the action that will best fit into his desired pattern of daily living.

In general terms the value of using a model based on functional assessment for care of the elderly has been well summarised by Panicucci (1983). She points out that most people (particularly the elderly) use functional ability to determine their health status rather than, or in spite of, the presence of specific pathology or disability. Also, a care plan with goal setting based on functional abilities helps the older person to work towards a desired pattern for daily living which takes account of any chronic disabilities, rather than leading him to believe all his health problems are treatable. A further asset of the model is its use of easily understood language (and everyday situations) which results in better communication between the members of the health team, the patient and his relatives/helpers.

However, the Roper model does require some additions in order to encompass all the facets of nutritional care. Chapman (1983) has demonstrated that it is not possible to make a valid assessment of functional problems associated with eating and drinking by a direct questioning method alone. In their introduction to the assessment of eating and drinking, Roper *et al.* (1981) state ' . . . Because most people enjoy talking about this Activity of Living, information about it is relatively easy to obtain'. The value of the information obtained by this method, however, is questionable, particularly in consideration of the care of the elderly. Most old people are only too anxious to provide those answers that they think are required by the interviewing nurse, and indeed often find it difficult to face up to problems that they may have. Roper's model also does not include specific consideration of physical and psychological factors relating to the problem. To overcome this modifications have been made, mainly in the way in which assessment is carried out. Data collected from the medical notes and by questioning the patient and relatives are supplemented by that from nonparticipant observation, which should be carried out in a structured manner to obtain specific information relating to nutritional status and nutritional problems, both actual and potential.

The elements of Roper's model for nursing

Roper's model focuses on Activities of Living (ALs). Twelve ALs are included in the model; maintaining a safe environment; communicating; breathing; eating and drinking; eliminating; personal cleansing and dressing; controlling body temperature; mobilising; working and playing; expressing sexuality; sleeping; and dying.

The basis for the model is that people who are in need of nursing care have some type of health-related problem, either actual or potential, which will in turn have an effect on the individual's everyday life, and hence on his ability to perform ALs. The ALs are used to provide a conceptual framework for the delivery of nursing care. They form the basis of assessment of the patient, to establish a picture of his normal lifestyle, and also to identify any problems that he may have, which may or may not be directly related to his particular health problem. These findings provide the necessary information to formulate a nursing care plan that is specifically tailored to the need of the individual.

This model provides an excellent framework for nursing care of elderly patients as its emphasis lies in the patient's daily life. Akhtar *et al.* (1973) define disability as being 'the inability to exist at home without help'. Using this definition, the prevalence of disability was found to rise from 12 per cent of the population aged 65 to 69, to more than 80 per cent in the population aged 85 years and over. In view of this observation, it is suggested that the use of a model that focuses on the individual's usual activities when not in hospital will provide relevant information for both short and long term plans. The details included in the assessment help to illuminate problems that are not directly related to the condition which caused the original hospitalisation. This must be to the patient's advantage as it provides the opportunity for the care team to examine these problems and possibly provide the necessary care/help to overcome them prior to the patient's discharge. It also provides a framework for assessment of all self-help capabilities. A decision that the patient is unable to return to the community and will require long term nursing care is based on this.

The main theme of this model therefore is to examine the effect of the health care problem(s) on the patient's daily life. This makes it suitable as a framework for the provision of nutritional care. It is also stressed that the ability to eat and drink not only has a direct bearing on the patient's capacity to overcome his health problem, but also provides the individual with the necessary fuel to carry out all the other ALs, and thus 'to exist at home without help'.

In order to focus on just one aspect of nursing care, nutritional care, it is necessary to adapt the model slightly. At the assessment stage, when details of ALs are collected, consideration of the possible relationship between each AL and the ability to eat and drink will be made. In addition to collecting data by direct questioning, further information will be recorded about physical status: the model as it stands does not directly focus on the physiological problems that a patient may have, and in nutritional care these are of obvious importance. This information (e.g. the presence of anaemia, diabetes, specific dietary related disorders) should be ascertained by the nurse both by direct measurement of the patient (height, weight) and also from consultation with the medical staff and from the patient's medical notes. Non-participant observation of the patient at mealtimes will also be included in the assessment to determine accurately the nature of the problems experienced under normal circumstances. The use of non-participant observation as a method of obtaining assessment information is prompted by research (Chapman 1983), which demonstrates that direct questioning and simulated testing alone are inadequate methods of obtaining reliable information on the individual's functional capacity to eat and drink. Patient interviews about nutritional problems revealed that the replies tended to be those that the patient thought were wanted. While a patient may be very willing to discuss the topic of food, when he is faced with food he may show no interest in it at all. The willingness to talk was a function of the need for company.

Similarly, it was found that some patients were unwilling or embarrassed to report that they had problems such as difficulty in cutting food, or with ill-fitting dentures, but on observation these became apparent. Furthermore, if a patient reports a difficulty during questioning, then an observation assessment can generally pinpoint the real nature of the problem and indicate the most appropriate course of action; for example, if weakness of one hand makes the manipulation of cutlery difficult, this may be overcome by the use of adapted cutlery, plate guards or a change in the type of food selected.

An illustration of the adapted model in use follows. The Patient Assessment Form and the Activities of Daily Living Form are as devised by Roper *et al.* (1983); in addition, a Nutritional Assessment Form is included bringing together all the assessment information obtained from the different sources.

Fig. 1.1 Patient assessment form: biographical and health data

Date of admission 4 Feb (16.00 hr.)	**Date of assessment** 5 Feb	**Nurse's signature** N. Jones

	Surname GREEN	**Forenames** HAROLD

Male [✓] **Age** [76] **Prefers to be addressed as**
Mr. Green

Female [ ] **Date of birth** 05.10.08

Single/Married/Widowed/Other

Address of usual residence   14 Church Street, Tadchester

Type of accommodation   2 bedroomed terrace house with upstairs WC/bathroom,
(incl. mode of entry if   steep staircase, 2 stairs down to kitchen
relevant)

Family/Others at this residence   none

Next of kin   **Name** REGINALD GREEN   **Address**   26 Clifford Road
                                                      Tadchester

Relationship son   **Tel. no.**   123456

Significant others **(incl. relatives/dependents** **visitors/helpers** **neighbours)** **Support services**	Relatives:– Helpers:– Visitors:– Services:–	one son, married, 2 grandchildren 8 & 10 yrs home help (for 3 yrs, 3 mornings a week) Mrs Clark friend, Jack Barnes, 2 evenings per wk, to play cards Meals on Wheels 5 × per wk Mon–Fri

Occupation   Retired (was self employed domestic carpenter)

Religious beliefs and relevant practices   C/E non-practising

Significant life crises   widowed 13 months ago (was married for 41 years)

Patient's perception of current health status
knows that he has had a 'stroke'

Family's perception of patient's health status
knows that he has had a 'stroke'

Reason for admission
For rehabilitation & subsequent assessment

Medical information (e.g. diagnosis, past history, allergies)
L. CVA residual R arm/face weakness
No past history of note
Never been in hospital before

GP Address Tel. no.	**Consultant Address Tel. no.**

Plans for discharge
Aim to discharge home, if possible.

Fig. 1.1 (continued)
Assessment of activities of living   Date

AL	Usual routines What he/she can and cannot do independently	Patient's problems (actual/potential) (p) = potential
• Maintaining a safe environment	finds stairs at home difficult second stairrail would help	lacks confidence with stairs
• Communicating	shy, withdrawn, embarrassed by slurred speech no comprehension problems with written or spoken word	slurred speech
• Breathing	normal, no problems, resps 18 per min non smoker	
• Eating and drinking	little interest in food since wife died problem using cutlery (weak R. hand) problem using cup, some dysphagia	see nutritional assessment
• Eliminating	continent of urine & faeces—uses a bottle at night nocturia × 2. Reports constipation (1 × 3 days) since wife died (**previously daily motion**)	constipation ? diet related
• Personal cleansing and dressing	dependent for shaving, denture cleaning & dressing (likes to look smart) Prior to stroke could manage, had a bath 1 × a week when son visited	dependent for washing & dressing
• Controlling body temperature	temp 36° on admission, within normal range no problems keeping warm house has central heating	
• Mobilising	R. sided weakness affecting balance. No paralysis of legs, though feels unsteady	loss of confidence in walking
• Working and playing	main hobby: making (+ selling via son) wooden toys enjoys T.V. newspapers, cards, dominos	loss of ability for hobby
• Expressing sexuality	nil of relevance	
• Sleeping	usually sleeps 11.30 pm–6 am. No medication makes tea at 6 am & returns to bed, with radio, until 8.30 am	
• Dying		

Fig. 1.2 Nutritional assessment form

Patient's name	Age	Date of admission	Date of assessment	Nurse's signature
Harold GREEN	76	4 Feb	6 Feb	N. Jones

PROBLEMS IDENTIFIED FROM A.L. ASSESSMENT

1. loss of use of R. hand (R. handed)
2. slurred speech
3. mild dysphagia
4. balance problems when walking
5. little interest in food
6. constipated

DAILY EATING PATTERN

Source of information patient

6 am   tea
9 am   tea, 2 pieces bread + marmalade
1 pm   M on W (M–F). Meal from or with son at we/ends
8 pm   tea cake and/or biscuits
6.30 pm   sandwich or boiled egg, biscuits
10 pm   milk drink

                            ? low Vit C
Calories: adequate   **Nutrients:** low roughage

PHYSICAL ASSESSMENT (using medical notes)

overall appearance light (? underweight)
height 172 cm   **reported wt.** 65 kg   **actual wt.** 60.2 kg
skin appearance dry, pale
mouth dry lips, buccal cavity clean
dentition full dentures   **fit of dentures** poor
anaemia yes (iron supplement prescribed)
other medical notes:

MEALTIME OBSERVATION

date 6 Feb   **meal** lunch
glasses worn yes /no̶   **dentures worn** yes /no̶
location at bedside
interest in meal little shown
use of cutlery difficulty—one handed did not try meat
transfer of food from plate to mouth some difficulty
amount eaten – main course potato only
                            – dessert half mousse only

use of cup managed
enjoyment of eating very little if any
other observations: obviously frustrated by inability to manage—seemed concerned that other patients may be watching him, spent most of time looking round. No dysphagia noted–but ate only mashed potato and mousse

SUMMARY Problems:

1. lack use R. hand
2. ? dysphagia
3. anaemia
4. disinterest in food
5. poor fitting dentures
6. constipation
7. dry lips
8. underweight/below reported weight

Observer N. Jones

Fig. 1.3 Nutritional care plan

Date   6 Feb

First evaluation after 1 week
Second evaluation after 3 weeks

Problem	Short term goal	Long term goal	Intervention	Evaluation
anorexic underweight lacks interest in food	demonstrate an interest in food	establish an 'adequate'* daily eating pattern	1 small, well presented, easily digested meals 2 encourage eating, offer verbal support when possible 3 when settled on ward arrange O.T. cookery classes	1/52 appetite improving taking more interest in food 3/52 attends and enjoys classes, now eager to learn
R. hemiplegia	demonstrate more active use of left hand	retrain R. hand	1 ask physio. for advice 2 reinforce & encourage exercises	1/52 enjoying exercise regimes though still feeling hampered at mealtimes 3/52 more confident, encouraged by slow increase of power to R. hand
can't cut food up has difficulty transferring food to mouth	demonstrate more active use of left hand	retrain R hand	1 provide an adapted knife/fork for L hand use 2 ensure an extra spoon is available 3 provide a nonslip mat and plate guard	1/52 adapted knife/fork and mat accepted, reluctant to use plate guard—further encouragement offered 3/52 now uses plate guard, as he realises that he isn't the only one with a problem
dry lips	moist lips, intact skin	improve hydration	1 vaseline for lips 2 encourage fluids	1/52 with increased fluids the problem is resolving
poor fitting dentures	no slippage experienced	improve fit or new dentures	1 try Grip Fix/denture cushions 2 refer to dentist	1/52 Grip Fix found to help 3/52 seen by hospital dentist recommended to see own dentist on discharge for new dentures

* 1. see Table 1.1 for DHSS recommended daily intakes

Fig. 1.3 (continued)

Problem	Short term goal	Long term goal	Intervention	Evaluation
some dysphagia	no discomfort on swallowing		discussion with patient when menu card is filled in, offer guidance regarding food that is easily swallowed	1/52 through trial and error found food that he could manage 3/52 dysphagia resolved
iron deficiency anaemia	blood picture within normal limits	to establish improved eating habits encourage iron rich foods	1 iron supplement until anaemia resolved 2 encourage selection of iron rich foods	1/52 anaemia resolving 3/52 Hg. within normal range, supplement reduced selection of iron rich foods continuing
little interest and ability in preparing foods		stimulate interest & skill development	refer to O.T. for cookery lessons	3/52 enjoys sessions made 'one handed' scones which he proudly shared with other patients
constipation	no constipation	restore previous bowel habit—daily after breakfast	1 suppositories/enema if required 2 high fibre diet add bran to soup/cereal (up to 20 g/day)	2 glycerine suppositories given with good result 3/52 excellent results with high bran diet, optimum level 15g/day some flatulence experienced with 20 g patient administers own bran b.d. in a cup of soup.
underweight	improved appetite	achieve weight increase consultant geriatrician to advise re target weight	1 well presented meals 2 food supplements if meals not eaten 3 teach food values and help in selection of foods	1/52 appetite improving enjoys Complan at night 3/52 attending cookery classes weight gain 1 kg now 61.2 kg

History

Mr. Green, a 76 year old retired self-employed carpenter, was admitted via the Accident and Emergency department to Prince Charles Ward, a 26 bed elderly assessment and rehabilitation unit, in the local District General Hospital.

He had suffered a stroke and had been found conscious, but slumped in a chair by Mrs. Hall, the lady who delivered his Meals on Wheels. Mrs. Hall called an ambulance and also notified Mr. Green's son, who was able to accompany him to hospital. On admission he appeared calm, but very withdrawn. He had been reassured that he would recover.

Prince Charles Ward is a purpose-built unit with beds arranged in four bays of six beds each, together with two side rooms for very ill patients. New arrivals are generally admitted into the first bay, and promoted to bays further away from the nurses' station as their rehabilitation progresses. The final bay has been nicknamed 'home-base' and has a sitting area and facilities for making tea and coffee, and low beds, rather than standard hospital beds. There is a large sitting room area on the ward which contains a well stocked library cabinet, together with games and cards, in addition to a radio and television. At one end of the sitting room are four tables, each seating up to four patients at meal times. The tables are covered with bright plastic coated fabric and whenever possible a small vase of flowers is placed on each one. Although the hospital operates a plated meals service, each patient wishing to eat at a table is encouraged to remove his cutlery and food from the tray before eating, to help to create a more normal eating atmosphere. The aim of the ward is to rehabilitate patients to return home, and this aim has been reflected in both the design and furnishing of the ward.

Mr. Green was admitted to a bed in the first bay (his nursing care and progress are discussed in the following sections). During his third week in hospital he was moved to a bed adjacent to his friend Mr. Brown in the third bay. A fortnight later both gentlemen moved into 'home-base' and after a further fortnight both men were discharged home.

Teaching and management implications

Nutritional care has many aspects, physical, physiological, psychological and social. It is important in formulating a care plan, and in subsequent review, to keep a realistic perspective on the goals to be achieved, that is to identify the problems in order of priority. For example, a patient admitted in a state of dehydration and severely cachectic obviously requires fluids and nourishment before starting care aimed at improving motivation towards self-help.

Ordering the priorities with Mr. Green for his care was not easy. It was obvious that he had a physical dysfunction (weak right hand) which made the actual task of eating and drinking difficult: however, in the early part of his rehabilitation programme this was compounded by acute embarrassment making him reluctant to attempt to eat as he was afraid of making a fool of himself.

Additionally, in the care of the elderly it should be remembered that to stimulate the appetite some nourishment needs to be taken, i.e. generally the more food that is eaten (within reason) the greater will be the desire for food. The success of this principle has been proved (Bastow *et al.* 1983) in the care of malnourished patients lacking the will to eat, by feeding them high calorie, nourishing supplements via a fine bore nasogastric tube overnight and then encouraging patients to eat as much as they desire during the day. The patient's appetite and desire to eat improved rapidly.

It is also pointed out that the model adheres to the philosophy of goal setting and regular evaluation. This format is particularly suitable for care planning and review with the patient since it has been shown (Panicucci 1983) that, particularly in the field of rehabilitation, patient compliance/adherence to care is better when the patient is involved with these stages of his care. This makes the model well suited to planning care for elderly people, as the emphasis of their care is on rehabilitation, either to allow for discharge or to achieve the optimum quality of life in long term care, if that is where they are to remain.

The approach adopted provided a framework for evaluation by comparing expected outcomes (short and long term goals incorporated into the care plan) with actual outcomes. This comparison demonstrated whether the care plan had been realistic and regular evaluation offered the opportunity to modify and update the care given and the nature of the anticipated goals. The use of a functional assessment model encourages the patient to be involved in his own care and monitor his progress in terms of his ability to perform those tasks which make him a functionally independent person.

It was decided at the outset of care planning that, in common with the majority of the patients on the ward, Mr. Green should be encouraged to take an active part in his management. Care plans were stored at the end of the bed, and daily goals and care alterations were decided jointly by the ward staff and the patient. Reporting took the form of a ward round, rather than a discussion at the nurses' station. Mr. Green, like many of the patients, found this rather strange at first. He had had no previous experience of being in hospital but had presumed that while on the ward almost all the decision making would be done for him. He took a few days to accept this approach, although by his third day on the ward he had begun to contribute to the daily planning meeting with all the nursing staff around his bed. As the days progressed his confidence grew and often he would be prepared for the discussion, having written (with difficulty, using his left hand) certain suggestions or points about his care which he wished the nurses to consider.

During the first few days of his stay Mr. Green's care centred on verbal encouragement; the trained staff spent several sessions sitting and talking with Mr. Green so that the real nature of his anxieties could be identified. It became apparent that with little experience of hospital or indeed of anyone who had suffered a stroke, Mr. Green thought that his problems were unique. A simple and most effective remedy to this problem was available. On the ward was Mr. Brown, a patient who had also suffered a stroke which had resulted in the loss of function of his right arm. Mr. Green was asked by the ward sister whether he would like to be introduced to Mr. Brown. They met and rapidly became good friends. The two men shared many interests and both enjoyed playing cards and dominoes, which helped to pass the time. Observing the two men together, the nurses noted that they were sharing ways of overcoming their difficulties and with this in mind, it was arranged that they should attend physiotherapy and occupational therapy sessions together, in order to encourage each other both during therapy and afterwards on the ward.

When evaluating Mr. Green's care it became apparent that by overcoming his social isolation, many of his other problems were solved at the same time. Mr. Green's interest in food increased, together with his manual dexterity, and power slowly returned to his right hand. Although full function was not restored prior to discharge, Mr. Green's motivation enabled him to use the available power to the full. At the first assessment some dysphagia was noted, but it was soon obvious that this was psychological rather than physiological. Mr. Green used difficulty in swallowing as an excuse not to eat. As his confidence and self esteem were restored, his appetite increased and the dysphagia ceased to be a problem. Ill-fitting dentures were dealt with by encouraging the use of a denture fixative. It was suggested that following discharge Mr. Green should visit his own dentist to arrange for a new set to be made as his current set were 15 years old and not surprisingly, the contours of his mouth had altered in that time. Also of great concern to Mr. Green was constipation. The establishment of good bowel habits by the addition of bran to his diet and the withdrawal of the regular use of laxatives required considerable encouragement by the nursing staff for the first few days of the new regime. However, as soon as Mr. Green was able to appreciate the improvement in his bowel habit, he was delighted and quickly took over the administration of his bran. He found the most palatable way to take it was in a cup of soup or meat extract twice a day.

On several occasions during Mr. Green's stay in hospital, his son was invited to join conversations between Mr. Green and members of the caring team (particularly nursing staff and the occupational therapist) so that future plans could be discussed. It was felt desirable to involve Mr. Green's family so as not to overwhelm him with the need to remember so many new practices.

Critique of the model in use

It must be remembered that a model only provides a framework for care and therefore invites adaptation. Roper herself suggests that a model can be used as a growing point for further thinking. Crow (1981) adds weight to this argument by pointing out that to date there is little recorded evidence that these theoretical frameworks have been validated.

> One danger nursing must not fall into is that of treating any one of these speculative models as dogma. This means that they must not be used as doctrines which are asserted as authoritative. It is essential that, in contrast, they always remain open to criticism and discussion. (Crow 1981)

In this section, it is intended to examine critically the use of Roper's theoretical framework to cope with a particular aspect of care, both in terms of general principles and the modification demonstrated in this chapter.

Bevis (1982) suggests that nurses are beginning to value the concept of holism. This philosophy proposes that a human being is an organismic whole, who cannot be treated as separate parts. However, Roper's work does not seem to reflect this, since she takes a reductionist view by presenting Man as a collection of Activities of Living. A further limitation of the Roper model is highlighted by Hodkinson (1981) who says that to perform an adequate assessment of an elderly person, biological, sociological and psychological factors need to be considered. Although Roper and her colleagues attempt to give guidance in these areas, there is a definite emphasis on biological elements.

The care plan format highlights other difficulties. There is evidence to suggest that it is used as a check list by the uninitiated, who lack the knowledge and skills for its intended application. In addition, the order in which the Activities of Living are presented may imply a priority. Although Roper makes it quite clear that this is not the case, the user may be tempted simply to work his or her way down the list. This point is of particular importance in the field of elderly care, where by tradition, a high proportion of staff have minimal nursing training, i.e. auxiliaries and assistants.

According to Roper *et al.* the assessment should focus around the individual's ability to carry out the 12 Activities of Living. The authors also suggest that it may not always be necessary to assess all activities. However, Aggleton and Chalmers (1985) point out 'some assessment of each is necessary before a nurse can safely ignore any of them'. It will be observed from Mr. Green's assessment that the areas of sexuality and dying received scant attention. Roper (1981) also reflects this approach. It is inevitable that differences of opinion will be expressed regarding this. In the final analysis, the decision rests with the professional nurse who is involved with the patient at the time.

Basically, this model focuses on the behavioural manifestations of fundamental human needs. The value of this when applied to nutritional care is that it relies on observable, measurable phenomena. A person's nutritional status is, in the truest sense, a product of the physical actions of ingestion and digestion. The focus therefore is on the individual's abilities to eat and drink appropriate nutrients and will give the person with a nutritional problem the best chance of improving his nutritional status. This was the case with Mr. Green.

The adaptation may appear lengthy, with considerable paperwork at the assessment stage. It must be stressed, however, that the length has been dictated by the minimum amount of information required to make a reliable assessment. It is intended that the adaptation is only used when a nutritional problem is identified and it will act as an insurance that all the relevant information is collected. As demonstrated earlier, there is evidence that lack of attention in this area of care leads to the unsatisfactory result of a poorly nourished patient. Again, it must be emphasised that the tool will only be as good as the individual using it. The need for relevant education for professional staff and in-service programmes for untrained personnel cannot be overestimated.

In conclusion, the adapted model provided a sound basis for planning care with a patient who had health problems directly affecting his nutritional status. It has been pointed out that models are not designed to be static but to be moulded and adapted as real life demands. This chapter has presented such an adaptation, which arose from the need to assess the nutritional status of an individual, by modifying a Model of Nursing based on functional assessment in a new way.

References

Aggleton P & Chalmers H 1985 Roper's Activities of Living Model. *Nursing Times*, 81, 7: 59–61.

Akhtar AJ, Broe GA, Crombie A *et al* 1973 Disability and dependency in the elderly at home. *Age and Ageing*, 2:102.

Bastow MD, Rawlings J & Allison SP 1983 Benefits of supplementary tube feeding after fractured neck of femur: a randomised controlled trial. *British Medical Journal*, 287: 1589–1592.

Beck ME 1977 *Nutrition and dietetics for nurses*. Churchill Livingstone, Edinburgh.

Bevis EMO 1982 *Curriculum building in nursing: a process*. C. V. Mosby Co., St. Louis.

Bloom A 1981 *Toohey's medicine for nurses*. Churchill Livingstone, Edinburgh.

Chapman EJ 1983 *Development of methods for the nursing assessment of the nutritional status of hospitalised*

elderly patients. Nursing Practice Research Unit.

Crow R 1981 Frontiers of nursing in the 21st century: development of models and theories on the concept of nursing. *Journal of Advanced Nursing*, 7: 111–116.

Cuthbertson DP 1932 Observations on the disturbance of metabolism produced by injury to the limbs. *Quarterly Journal of Medicine*, 1: 233–246.

Davidson S 1975 *Human nutrition and dietetics*. Churchill Livingstone, Edinburgh.

DHSS 1969 *Report on public health* (Medical Subjects No. 120). HMSO, London.

Evans E & Stock AL 1971 Dietary intakes of geriatric patients in hospital. *Nutrition and Metabolism*, 13: 21–35.

Hector W 1980 *Modern nursing, theory and practice*. Heinemann, London.

Hodkinson HM 1981 *An outline of geriatrics*. Academic Press Inc., London.

Older MJW, Edwards E & Dickerson JWT 1980 A nutrient survey in elderly women with femoral neck fractures. *British Journal of Surgery*, 67: 884–886.

Panicucci CL 1983 Functional assessment of the older adult in the acute care setting. *Nursing Clinics of North America*, 18, ii: 355–363.

Pearce E 1975 *A general textbook of nursing*. Faber & Faber, London.

Roper N, Logan WW & Tierney AJ 1980 *The elements of nursing*. Churchill Livingstone, Edinburgh.

Roper N, Logan WW & Tierney AJ 1981 *Learning to use the process of nursing*. Churchill Livingstone, Edinburgh.

Roper N, Logan WW & Tierney AJ 1983 *Using a model for nursing*. Churchill Livingstone, Edinburgh.

Vir S & Love AHG 1976 Nutritional status of institutionalised and non-institutionalised aged in Belfast, Northern Ireland. *American Journal of Clinical Nutrition*, 32: 1934–1947.

2

A positive step towards independence: self-medication using Orem's Self-care model

Ann Bergen

Introduction

The link between nursing practice and nursing knowledge is a theme to which Dorothea Orem (1980) devotes a considerable amount of discussion and elaboration. She argues that, in order to deliver effective care, practice should proceed from knowledge, which describes and explains the concepts underlying the helping service of nursing. Of the varying degrees of generality of nursing knowledge, that which can be applied to all instances of nursing forms its basic theory. And, she says, 'the mastery of a general, comprehensive theory of what nursing is and why nursing is produced and supported by social groups is a first step for nurses who want to be aware of the relationship between what they know and what they do as nurses'.

This concern, expressed by the nurse theorist, that nursing actions be built on a well grounded theoretical infrastructure, is one which is echoed by the practitioner at the grass roots; indeed, it is this practitioner who is in the best position to test the viability of various theories in relation to standards of care. The following discussion is an attempt to analyse how one compelling issue within nursing care of the elderly—a failure to take prescribed medication correctly—was tackled with reference to Orem's own 'concepts of practice', which emphasise self-care.

The discussion opens with an investigation of the problem in question—how it is defined, its extent and possible causes and methods of reducing it. The focus is then narrowed to a consideration of one elderly person and her particular difficulties with managing her drugs, and Orem's model of self-care is offered as an appropriate framework to support consequent nursing action. There follows a more detailed study of the model with a parallel account of the patient's actual care set out within the stages of the nursing process. Finally, both model and care are re-analysed in the light of how effectively they related to, and informed, each other. Difficulties arising are presented, along with possible reasons, and the rationales behind amendments considered necessary.

Note: The care plan, featured in Appendices II and III, is necessarily selective, illustrating only aspects considered relevant to the main theme, and shown at one point in time. An attempt has been made to preserve the 'holistic' approach by retaining interconnected problems, without becoming overwhelmed by the well-known phenomenon of multipathology in old age.

The problem: non-compliance among elderly drug takers

Definitions

The problem of elderly patients taking (or not taking) prescribed drugs has to date been studied largely from the medical viewpoint and the concept of 'non-compliance' has, over the last few years, firmly entered the vocabulary of medical literature (Haynes *et al.* 1979). Yet, even within authoritative circles, there is no agreed definition of the term or, consequently, any one method of calculating its extent, determinants or remedies with regard to this particular clientele.

To Norton (1982) compliance 'refers to the circumstances in which the behaviour of the patient is controlled by the physician' and 'may be an all-or-none affair or a matter of degree'. This approach has been criticised, not least by nurses (Potter 1981, Moughton 1982), on the grounds of its moral overtones and its assumption that patients should always obey the professional. Only differing in degree is the interpretation put forward by Haynes *et al.* (1979) as 'simply the extent to which a person's behaviour. . . . coincides with medical or health advice'. Here, 'adherence' and 'compliance' are seen as interchangeable terms, but this would appear to be a mere semantic manoeuvre in order to minimise the judgemental connotation.

A contrasting definition emphasises the 'negotiation' aspect in compliance. It is, say Given and Given (1984), 'the result of the individual's interaction with providers and others in his environment', and Moughton (1982) goes as far as suggesting the term 'contracting' be used instead of 'complying'. This redefinition of relationships (significantly, by nurses) has relevance for the nurse seeking both suitable models and appropriate strategies to promote compliant behaviour.

But compliance has also a more specific definition with regard to drug taking. Smith and Andrews (1983) refer to the 'compliance percentage' in calculating the extent of deviation from a known drug schedule:

$$\text{compliance} \% = \frac{\text{number of tablets used since discharge}}{\text{number of tablets prescribed for period}} \times 100.$$

This is of greatest importance in trials, where specificity is essential and where non-compliance may be defined as a particular percentage of over- or under-dosage. Other more general (but nevertheless useful) interpretations vary from any error in dosage or timing (Kent and Dalgleish

1983) to where deviation from the regime is sufficient to interfere with the achievement of the therapeutic goal (O'Hanrahan and O'Malley 1981). As the first is as significant to nurses as the second in its potential to endanger health, the prescription for care must be the same.

Before leaving the subject of definition, one more area of debate should be highlighted. Macdonald and Macdonald (1982) criticise Haynes' definition as being too wide and contend that the term 'non-compliance' should be limited to factors over which the patient has control. This would seem to be of less service to nurses than the more inclusive definition, in view of the many factors underlying patient responses (considered below) amenable to intervention. The differentiation made by Parkin *et al.* (1976) between failure to understand (non-comprehension) and understanding but failure to follow instructions (non-compliance) is useful only insofar as it directs remedial action. Thus, the concept of non-compliance for this purpose is taken to be characterised by a breakdown in the nurse-patient 'contracting' system, resulting in any deviation from a prescribed (drug) regimen, and attributable to any cause.

Incidence

Definitions are, of course, only part of the appreciation of any problem. Its overall extent and particular preponderance in certain population samples studied need to be identified prior to the application of research findings and/or theoretical models.

The Royal College of Physicians in 1984 highlighted the disproportionate prescribing of medication for the elderly, but earlier studies came to similar conclusions. Christopher *et al.* (1978) in a cross-sectional, one day ward study of 873 patients aged 65 and over, found the average individual to be taking 3.3 drugs (4 on geriatric wards) and 15% to be taking 10 or more. Williamson's much more ambitious, multi-centre study in the same year found 81.3% of the over 65 s to be taking drugs, with 25.9% taking 4–6 in number. Community studies are no less striking. Law and Chalmers (1976) conducted a general practice survey which (though now a little dated) yielded a regular treatment prevalence of 87% for those aged 75 plus. 34% were taking 3–4 drugs a day. A more recent trial by Kiernan and Isaacs (1981) differentiated regular, occasional, prescribed and non-prescribed medicines, of which the total average taken was 4.3 a day.

One corollary of this therapeutic enthusiasm, pinpointed by the Royal College, is the high non-compliance rate among the elderly and the potentially serious results of this. Parkin *et al.* (1976) found that 66 of 130 patients followed up on discharge (50.8%) were not taking their drugs correctly, while Wandless and Davie (1977) also put the number of non-compliers at over half. According to Macdonald *et al.* (1977) the figure (based on the control group of their sample) could be as high as 75%, again noted by the Royal College. One exception to these findings is that of Smith and Andrews (1983), in whose general practice sample 92% were over 95% compliant. However, because of the number studied (35), it cannot be taken as representative and, as the authors state, the 'Hawthorne effect' (Roethlisberger and Dickson 1939) could also have operated to sway the results. It is, therefore, now well substantiated that non-compliance among elderly drug takers is a significant problem.

Causes

The determinants, as well as the magnitude, of any problem must be calculated before care plans can be drawn up and implemented. Since, in the process of nursing, 'nurses and patients act together to allocate the roles of each' (Orem 1980), the focus here will be placed on those studies indicating causal links with the patient-practitioner relationship, or with the patient himself, where such a relationship may mitigate the problem. In other words, such lines of enquiry as demographic data (age, sex, class, educational level), the nature of the patient's disease or of the drug regimen will not be touched on; these characteristics are only indirectly, if at all, amenable to nursing influence.

Many analyses of non-compliance look at the psychological attributes of groups of respondents, attributes such as mental functioning, facility for understanding, knowledge, memory and established attitudes and perceptions. The first of these can be assessed in the elderly through instruments such as that devised by Qureshi and Hodkinson (1974). Swift (1982), in his review of the literature, concluded that it was not an influential factor, though Shannon (1983), in a nursing trial, found that those scoring low on the questionnaire were less likely to follow guidelines. Macdonald and Macdonald (1982) came to similar conclusions.

Where knowledge and understanding have been put under the microscope, conclusions are generally drawn from the impact which the introduction of information-giving has had on the trial outcome. Here, findings are conflicting. Parkin *et al.* (1976) found that knowledge of the disease bore little relation to consequent behaviour and Macdonald and Macdonald (1982) substantiated this. With respect to knowledge of treatment, under half of the patients surveyed by Kiernan and Isaacs (1981) knew the names of their drugs, and less knew the purpose of prescribed than non-prescribed medicines. But even knowledge cannot correlate necessarily with desired response. In the Parkin study, though 46 of the 130 did not understand their regimen, 20 of the remaining 84 understood but still did not follow instructions. Part of the reason could be poor recall of instructions or advice (Atkinson *et al.* 1978), though Hogue (1979) suggests the crucial element is 'not only knowledge per se but also knowledge of the way the patient defines his situation'.

One approach which takes patient perceptions into account is the Health Belief Model, described by Becker *et al.* (1979) as a framework for explaining the likelihood of a person carrying out recommended (preventive) health action. Briefly, it hinges on his calculations of the relative benefits and disadvantages of such actions. These will depend partly on the way in which the health message is communicated by the professional and, suggest Given and Given (1984), the individual's resultant feeling of self control. It is an attractive theoretical construct for explaining drug-taking behaviour, since within it can be subsumed such factors as the 'defaulter' who is 'feeling better', so ceases to take his therapy, or the way a high-involvement profile on the part of the practitioner appears to promote compliance (Hulka 1979, Smith and Andrews 1983). It may even account for the surprising lack of consensus as regards the role played by side- and secondary effects (Haynes *et al.* 1979 versus Norton 1982), if being forewarned promotes willingness. Whether it does or not, it is clear that the causes of non-compliance need careful assessment; they are not only diverse and very individual, but usually not attributable to any single reason (O'Hanrahan and O'Malley 1981).

Improving compliance

Strategies aimed at improving compliance fall broadly into two (though not exclusive) categories. Firstly, there are those trials focusing on, and aiming to modify, the psychological attributes referred to above through some programme of teaching. And secondly, there have been efforts to build on this by increasing the individual's self-control through a scheme of client-managed therapy.

Mental functioning is not effectively subject to manipulation, though Atkinson *et al.* (1977) remind us that as 'intellectual impairment is not caused by old age', one should not automatically underestimate the ability of the elderly. Level of knowledge on the other hand can be increased, as with a younger individual, through appropriately used drug-taking manuals and protocols (American Society of Hospital Pharmacists 1978, Weibert and Dean 1980, Smith 1977, Barofsky 1977). Finally, memory can be prompted using certain aids, though choice of type will depend on the individual; Macdonald *et al.* (1977) found that 'counselling' reduced errors by a third and that this was effective even for poorly orientated patients. Crome *et al.* (1980) tested the 'Dosett Box', while Lundin *et al.* (1980) compared oral, written and supplementary aids in variable combinations. Wandless and Davie's (1977) classic trial on similar lines suggested, as did Davidson's

(1974), that a calendar-type reminder was most successful.

Each of the programmes involved some element of learning theory which, as it relates to the elderly, involves certain special characteristics. For instance, 'older people work better at concrete, rather than abstract tasks' (Dall and Gresham 1982)—hence the very tangible aids—and 'older subjects take longer and want more information than the younger ones in order to achieve the same results' (Bromley 1974)—illustrated in the fact that most programmes extended over some weeks. But in addition, as Rosenberg (1976) states, 'the use of an educational process that involves patient participation in the decision making is the sine qua non for effective programming'. This philosophy forms the basis of self-medication trials.

An individual's health beliefs and attitudes are thought to be more readily changed through behavioural, rather than educational, strategies (Haynes 1976). In other words, modification of fundamental perceptions of a given situation by reinforcement, feedback and transfer of responsibility is often a better guarantee of subsequent actions than simple, fixed-content information giving. Shannon (1983) studied a group of elderly rehabilitation patients whose desired responses to drug teaching were rewarded by allowing self-management of the regimen. Her work involved 'counselling' patients one week prior to discharge with regard to their drugs, then providing them with two days' personalised supply that they would be responsible for holding and consuming. Drug taking behaviour was closely monitored and recorded and, if satisfactory, followed by a further three days' supply and less structured supervision. By discharge, the group were making significantly fewer discrepancies than the controls, who were 'counselled' only. The work was based on the similar trial of Baxendale *et al.* (1978) in Glasgow, while Roberts (1978) and Hatch and Tapley (1982) also undertook projects consistent in their findings.

Research evidence therefore suggests that compliance can be promoted by suitably planned nursing intervention and the subsequent discussion attempts to illustrate this through the application of one particular nursing model to one particular patient.

Rationale for choice of model

The patient

Miss Emily Jones was admitted to the acute/assessment ward for the elderly primarily on account of severe dyspnoea; she could walk no further than 100 yards (with a stick, due to arthritis) without becoming extremely distressed, presented with a productive cough and complained of disturbed sleep at night. A medical diagnosis of left heart failure, compounded by chronic obstructive airways disease, was put forward and the appropriate drug treatment (bronchodilators, steroids and diuretics) was started. Miss Jones was aware of the reason behind her admission ('to find out why I'm always short of breath') but the symptoms represented a deviation from her normal health status and lifestyle which upset her.

The patient lived in sheltered housing with a sister, Agnes, only a few years her junior. They were coping fairly well and had a very supportive warden, but nurses discovered in conversation that the patient had recently become rather 'forgetful' and her sister doubted if she had been taking her tablets regularly. In addition, the telltale signs of occasional 'accidents with the waterworks' were worrying and, after examination, an anticholinergic drug was added to her treatment. Both sisters were keen that their normal living arrangements should quickly resume, but that these problems should firstly be minimised as far as possible.

The model

Rehabilitation is 'the process whereby disabled individuals are provided with opportunities to develop skills necessary for optimum functioning' (Knust and Quarn 1983). It puts the onus as much on the client as the health professional to work towards this, emphasising what Orem (1980) describes as 'self-care'. Rehabilitation, in the sense of the withdrawal of nursing support

and management of/adjustment to the problems of breathing, memory loss and incontinence, was also the overall aim of care for Miss Jones. A major factor here was the control of disease by drugs, so there arose the specific need for the patient to learn, and become independent in, this aspect of her care.

To Orem (1980) 'nursing has as its special concern the individual's need for self-care action and the provision and management of it on a continuous basis in order to sustain life and health, recover from disease or injury and cope with their effects'. This philosophy agrees with the aims already outlined for the elderly person under consideration and therefore seemed a particularly apt model to use. Of course, Orem is not unique amongst nurse theorists in emphasising independence; Roy (1980) through adaptation, and Roper (1976) through promoting skills in the activities of living, also see the aim of nursing care in terms of health achieved by patient action and nurse support. But for Miss Jones, Roy's categories (modes) did not seem an obvious way of promoting the learning, knowledge and skills necessary to improve compliance. Nor was it immediately clear where to place drug-taking in Roper's 'AL' framework—a nurse may not reach the source of the problem within this model. It may also have been difficult to place the required nursing care within her preventing, comforting and dependent categories. Orem's less structured yet comprehensive format was therefore adopted as a guide to care.

The model in use

Self-care

The concept of self-care, which is central to Orem's model, is defined as 'the practice of activities that individuals initiate and perform on their own behalf in maintaining life, health and well-being' (Orem 1980). The 'self' component is taken to mean both 'for' (oneself) and 'given by' (oneself), although the term 'self-care agent' refers only to the latter (that is, the person taking action). Joseph (1980) comments that 'by approaching self-care practices in relation to both

Fig. 2.1   Orem's conceptual framework for nursing (Orem 1980)

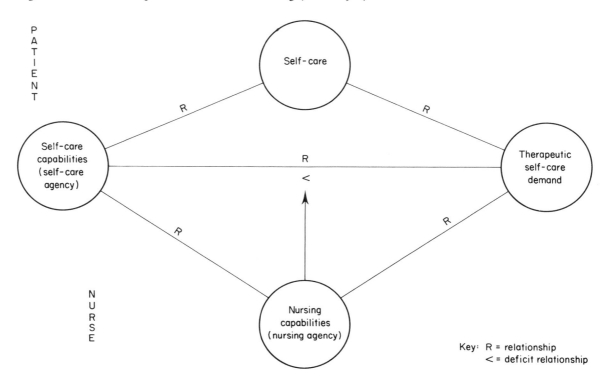

health and disease or illness, Orem includes the total health-illness spectrum in her framework'. This is useful in its ability to account for and promote behaviour taken in a preventive, as well as therapeutic, capacity (for instance, the drug-taking which Miss Jones would need to continue once the immediate symptoms had abated).

Orem's specific concept of self-care is further underpinned by a number of premises. It can, she believes, be achieved potentially by all human beings and this is effected through deliberate actions and learned behaviour. Once self-care requirements have been identified, ways to meet them necessarily follow. These 'technologies' or 'processes' vary between individuals and must be seen within the social and cultural contexts which produce them. The underlying assumption is, as Campbell (1984) points out, that self-care 'has to be based on knowledge rather than whim, enabling patients to make informed decisions about their care'.

Patient profile

Orem advocates a systematic approach to nursing in order to maximise individualised care. The basis of an individual's uniqueness is usually enshrined in a patient profile and, though Orem's account of the nursing process gives little guidance on the acquisition of these formal details, she does acknowledge that '. . . it is important for nurses to make initial observations about patients and their families in order to provide themselves with information they can use to guide their interactions and communications with patients' (Orem, 1980). Consequently, such a procedure was undertaken using standard documentation.

But, with the thrust of Miss Jones' therapeutic management being directed at a resumption of normal/optimal functioning, and her wish to return home to her sister, a profile format which included interpersonal details and aimed at community transfer within the self-care model was, ideally, called for. Reutter (1984) offers such a construct in the shape of a family assessment guide, combining family systems theory with Orem's self-care framework. The family, in Reutter's model, shows structural and functional components which have a bearing on both internal (the individual members) and external (its negotiation with wider social systems) aspects of health and integrity. If later evaluation suggested the original details were inadequate, this notion of family structure could be used to obtain additional baseline data pertaining to communication patterns, role relationships, power structure and value systems within the two-person household (a suggested pro forma is detailed in Appendix I). This would provide useful documented insight for later care planning in, for instance, gauging the degree of support with medication and incontinence management which could be expected from Agnes Jones, without risking role conflict and/or overload. With regard to function, however, as defined by Reutter, it would seem that this could more appropriately be assessed by incorporating it in the self-care requisites of the nursing assessment (see below) by giving them a group orientation. Finally, family perception of the health situation would be included as suggested by both Reutter (1984) and Joseph (1980), as a necessary prelude to care planning.

Assessment

Although Orem does not use the term 'assessment', she describes an 'investigative operation' leading to a nursing diagnosis, which can be regarded as synonymous with the more commonly used term (Aggleton and Chalmers 1985). Her equivalent to assets and needs, which form the basis of assessment, consists of a determination of (respectively) self-care abilities and self-care deficits and there are three basic stages in establishing these.

Firstly, because self-care has purpose, Orem analyses it in terms of self-care requisites (or requirements). There are three types:

Universal—based on the assumption that human beings have common needs which must be met in order to support life and functional and structural integrity. A 'checklist' of these is provided, covering aspects such as need for air, water, food, etc. Although Miss Jones was assessed on all these parameters, the documentation focuses on those relevant to the medication self-care issue (Appendix II).

Developmental—special needs occurring at different stages of development, from intrauterine to adult maturation. It could be argued that an elderly individual is no longer 'developing', in the sense of maturing. However, Orem's text stipulates that events or conditions which are usually age-associated also feature in this category. She states specifically that 'rehabilitation focuses on developmental self-care requisites associated with conditions resulting from pathology, medical diagnosis or treatment procedures, or the results of inadequate nursing or dependent care' (Orem 1980). Miss Jones' newly emerging need to cope with a drug schedule was one such case in point. It was however felt that 'age-related' or 'life-span' more accurately described these requisites than Orem's terminology.

Health-deviation—particular needs emerging when ill-health occurs, in order to prevent and/or regulate its effects. Again, selective criteria are illustrated (Appendix II) in connection with Miss Jones' breathing difficulties because of the interplay of this with drug-taking.

Secondly, nurses must conceptualise and identify the totality of self-care actions to be performed in order to meet known self-care requisites and Orem terms these 'self-care demands' or 'prescriptions for continuous self-care'. Significantly, they do not always emanate from the individual on whom the demand is made. A breakdown of Miss Jones' self-care requisites contained many demands which only emerged following negotiation between nurse and patient.

Thirdly, when self-care demands are known for individuals, the nurse must assess the agency (or ability)—actual or potential—available to meet them. This may centre on the individual herself or on family members. If any deficit occurs between a self-care demand and the ability to meet it, this forms the basis of a nursing diagnosis or problem. In addition, it is important to ascertain why this deficit exists and to examine the patient's level of knowledge, motivation and skills in the light of the demand they must fulfil. At this stage, it is important to verify that an inability to act independently does actually establish the basis of a problem, rather than merely a pre-existing potentiality for under-provision, which has been compensated for by an alternative. For instance, had Miss Jones' sister been more consistently (and willingly) involved in prompting and guidance with regard to toilet and medication, these particular self-care deficits would have been translated into dependent-care abilities (and therefore, not problems).

Nursing care planning

In Orem's model, the formulation of a care plan must be seen within her overall concept of the purpose of nursing. 'The condition that validates the existence of a requirement for nursing', she says, 'is the absence of the ability to maintain continuously that amount and quality of self-care which is therapeutic in sustaining life and health, in recovering from disease or injury or in coping with their effects' (Orem 1980). Designing and planning care are professional nursing and management operations and the plan forms 'the starting point for the primarily practical phase of the nursing process in which the patient (or family) is assisted in self-care matters to achieve identified and described health and health-related results' (ibid.). A number of premises underlie this phase of nursing, which can be illustrated with reference to Miss Jones' care plan, specifically as it relates to medication (Appendix III).

Firstly, nursing is an 'interaction' process between nurse and patient, with contractual and complementary characteristics—the 'acting together' in role allocation, noted above (and incidentally echoing Given and Given's contractual nature of compliance). Miss Jones' plan acknowledged this implicitly in its attention to patient motivation towards nursing (that is, self-care) goals, in its orientation towards patient responsibility and in the way the nurse-patient-sister relationship itself featured as a formal and structural component of care. Thus Miss Jones was highly motivated to 'get better' and the projected way of achieving this was through taking responsibility for medication. And the acceptance of nursing input allowed for a dynamic interplay of explanation, discussion, prioritisation, supervision and finally, nurse withdrawal.

Secondly, nursing is seen in terms of 'systems theory'. Orem defines a system as anything that can be viewed as a single, whole thing, which can be best understood by identifying the elements underlying its structure. Nursing, as a helping service, comprises three basic helping subsystems, within which the specific, discrete actions of nurses and patients take place. The wholly compensatory system is appropriate where the patient is unable to engage in deliberate actions and the nurse must act for him (as for the comatose patient). The partly compensatory system is operative when the nurse and patient both perform care measures with varying degrees of responsibility. The supportive-educative system occurs where the patient can learn to perform required measures relating to decision-making, behaviour control and the acquisition of knowledge and skills. This is the system of choice for multi-person units and rehabilitative nursing, where 'assisting through teaching must be adapted to age as well as to past education and experience' (ibid.). It was planned to use this particular self-care example for Miss Jones, combined with research-based strategies related to compliance. This entailed promoting responsible decision-making in drug selection (Given and Given 1984), behaviour control in 'shaping' towards compliance (Haynes 1976) and knowledge/skill acquisition through information-giving and practice (Rosenberg 1976).

Thirdly, in formulating courses of action for meeting patient self-care demands, nurses must select 'valid and reliable processes and technologies' (Orem 1980). This implies research- and theory-based interventions, instanced in this case not only by the foregoing, but also by the drug-counselling programme (Macdonald *et al* 1977), the timing geared toward the special needs of the elderly (Bromley 1974) and self-medication (Shannon 1983).

Implementation and evaluation

Orem's third phase of the nursing process involves intervention to regulate the therapeutic self-care demand and the self-care agency. Because of this regulatory nature of the nursing system, evaluation is seen as a logical extension of the same operation, rather than a separate entity. Thus, nursing performance and patient condition are documented (implementation), giving rise to evidence from which the relationship of the two can be assessed and forward recommendations made (evaluation). Evaluation therefore takes the form of (*i*) monitoring patients, and assisting them to monitor themselves, to determine the extent and effectiveness of self-care, and (*ii*) making judgements about the results of nursing performance in terms of patient wellbeing. But appraisal, as Aggleton and Chalmers (1985) stress, should always be stated in terms of patient achievement, rather than whether nursing intervention (which is likely to diminish over time, anyway) is carried out.

Implementing care for Miss Jones according to Orem's criteria did not take place without difficulties. In 'acting together', the nursing role often appeared easier to define than that of the patient, at least in the early stages, where drug administration was largely a nurse-initiated operation. However, the patient was a willing receiver of nursing input and her priority for care, which centred on the breathing difficulty, was relatively easy to respect because of its physical (and therefore obvious) manifestations.

The use of the supportive-educative mode presented a greater challenge. Discussing, supporting, teaching, guiding and enabling strategies, though acknowledged as relevant, were in practice often glossed over, probably because they constituted 'invisible' aspects of care. Most nurses needed as much encouragement and support as the patient to persevere with the selected approaches and the availability of a co-ordinator was a distinct advantage.

Research evidence was introduced through utilising principles, rather than by replication. This was largely governed by the constraints of the hospital setting. Shannon's (1983) model for self-medication, for instance, could not be reproduced fully, but its rationale of encouraging responsibility was applied through limited patient participation (Appendix III).

Formal evaluation of patient responses brought feedback for nurses, either reinforcing present strategies or prompting changes.

Where the move from a compensatory to a supportive-educative approach was made, it indicated not only an acceptance of the model in use, but also, indirectly, effective intervention. For instance, when Miss Jones' breathing difficulties improved with medication, it allowed her to concentrate on managing her own therapy, and the nurses to move to a facilitating role. In addition, it allowed her mobility level to improve to the extent that she was able to walk the distances required at home without breathlessness and this in turn led to greater independence in other activities. She also managed to regulate those activities within her breathing capacity.

This meant that becoming responsible and effective in drug-taking assumed priority, not only to maintain her health status but also to promote continence and a re-establishment of a normal and sufficiently independent lifestyle to enable a return home. Here, progress was not so clear cut. Motivation was less pressing, since absence of medication self-care did not present itself to the patient with the immediacy of a distressing physical symptom. Certainly, her ability improved in this area, but not uniformly; she could soon identify the times of day when drugs were due and cope with the actual mechanics of administration, but invariably failed to select the appropriate types and numbers of tablets or demonstrate any knowledge regarding names and actions. It was clear that the deficit between self-care demand and ability remained, and analysis of the situation identified three possible reasons for this:

1   Inadequate assessment. For instance, did the patient have the potential for achieving self-care in this area or was this aim unrealistic? Had it comprised all the factors indicated by research to be significant in non-compliance, including the piloting of potential aids?
2   Failure to produce a 'contractual' care plan. In retrospect, did the nurses really formulate goals and strategies with, rather than for, the patient?
3   Inconsistency in implementation. Were all the nurses sufficiently briefed in, and committed to, the approach?

These findings, it must be said, would have been due to the actual way an as yet unfamiliar model was realised, rather than the actual model per se. The bridge between theory and practice was proving a challenging one to cross. Yet in the last analysis, it was from the same theory, applied a little more pragmatically, that an amended and more effective plan emerged.

In the search for a plan which would at once comprehend and render practical Orem's ideals, the family systems theory of Reutter presented itself. Although not formalised in application, its principles did lead to a retrospective reassessment of independent functioning potential, which highlighted Orem's dependent-care concept. The proposition was put that if Miss Jones' sister had not been overtly involved in care or support to date, this did not necessarily indicate an unwillingness or inability to do so. Discussion, followed by teaching in medication-taking, began again, this time focusing on both Emily and Agnes as the self-care agency. This legitimised the involvement of a third party within the self-care framework, at the same time making up the deficit (of knowledge and skills) which the patient lacked. In addition, the introduction of a Dosett Box (Crome *et al.* 1980) allowed Miss Jones to maintain her existing capacity to cope with handling and timing.

The other two interrelated issues highlighted in the care plan were similarly incorporated into the emergent framework. Self-care demands for elimination were partially met as Miss Jones remembered (perhaps surprisingly) to go to the toilet fairly regularly during the day. This may have been due to 'cueing' by other patients or ward activities, but her parallel, successful timing with drugs lends credence to the supposition that the behaviour may have been nurse-initiated. Occupational and physiotherapists provided a new walking stick, raised toilet seat and dressing aids (for both hospital and home) which assisted access. Persistent occasional nocturnal incontinence led to a reformulation of nursing prescription such that her sister became involved in the provision of the anticholinergic drugs (via the Dosett Box), proper use of incontinence aids and occasional reminders to visit the toilet.

Finally, 'normal functioning', as a comprehensive self-care requisite, served as a general statement of desired function in other areas. The criterion for goal setting was broadened out so that the emphasis shifted from personal self-care abilities to effective family structure and function. The fact that this was retained facilitated the anticipated and desired discharge from hospital.

Critique of the model in use

The assessment of nursing models as used in particular care settings (termed 'summative evaluation' by Aggleton and Chalmers 1985) is important for its contribution to the development of a sound knowledge base for nursing. Yet, as Harper (1984) points out, few studies verify theoretical constructs of self-care and nursing systems at more than a conceptual framework level—this despite the need to develop substantive knowledge and skills in, for instance, medication self-care. Harper's own work partly offsets this deficit, while that of Knust and Quarn (1983) has applied and validated the self-care construct in the area of rehabilitation nursing.

With these guidelines in mind, the selection of Orem's model for Miss Jones' care would seem suitable, especially against the background of today's philosophy of self-reliance, prevention and holism in health matters. Yet, the advent of individualised patient care notwithstanding, nurses were slow in taking this philosophy on board, a drawback more likely attributable to unfamiliarity, as previously suggested, than to lack of integrity within the model. Orem's theories were, of course, conceived in the United States and to a certain extent reflect attitudes and values not yet widespread in Britain. Indeed, her terminology itself might sometimes sound obscure to a British audience, as Anna *et al.* (1978) and Iveson-Iveson (1982) have suggested, and only a close reading of her discussion of self-care establishes her individualised conception of it.

While the deficits in the formal database have been discussed, the overall assessment format led to a comprehensive and specific account of Miss Jones' problems. However, Butterfield (1983) has criticised Orem's concept of health (the aim of self-care) in that, like the World Health Organization's famous definition (1946), it is based on a unidirectional assumption that fails to accommodate anything less than complete well-being and movement towards this. Orem's notion of developmental self-care requisites illustrates the point, the implication being that maturity is a status constantly being aimed at. As suggested earlier, a change of terminology when considering the elderly might preserve the idea of emerging, age-related needs without the incongruent overtones.

Orem's criteria for planning nursing intervention seemed particularly relevant to the main themes of Miss Jones' care. Her 'contracting' ideal is in accord with the nursing definition of compliance, outlined above, with its emphasis on negotiation rather than mere obedience. It also stresses the importance of individual perception of health, as described in the Health Belief Model, a precondition of effective nurse-patient interaction and health care.

Implementing care based on the model presented the greatest challenge. Firstly, although Orem allows for dependent as well as self-care as a valid end in itself, this principle needed expanding before it could be fully utilised. Here Reutter's (1984) family systems theory offered

guidelines for adapting care to suit the elderly within an anticipated community setting. It involved a more comprehensive assessment of the components, structure and function of what became, in effect, a new and viable self-care unit.

Secondly, and following on from this, one might question the continuing relevance of Orem's model once Miss Jones had been discharged. Although Orem allows for different levels of nurse-patient interaction (dependent upon self-care capacity at any one time) nursing is actually restricted to that period when an imbalance exists between the individual's ability and the demand placed upon him. So, although Miss Jones returned home 'in balance' as it were, there would be no provision within the model of anything akin to a 'surveillance' plan, to monitor any potential breakdown in drug-taking behaviour. This may occur if, for instance, Miss Jones' sister herself became ill or infirm.

Thirdly, although medication self-care has been shown in many accounts to be a worthwhile undertaking, there are limits to the extent to which this can be carried out within the British hospital framework. Health Authority drug policies often err on the side of caution, when self-responsibility is seen to involve a certain amount of risk-taking by the patient, with the result that the nurse's autonomy is often called into question. This was why a limited degree of self-care only could be achieved with Miss Jones.

Finally, Orem's implementation-evaluation continuum proved useful in the final phase of the nursing process, since it emphasised its dynamic nature. It allowed a degree of flexibility which meant that initial goals could be restated when nursing intervention failed to lead to desired results. Indeed, the whole structure proved—rightly or wrongly—adaptable to the particular need. Such feedback, in turn, facilitated summative evaluation, the importance of which was outlined earlier.

Aggleton and Chalmers (1985) comment that nursing models should not be seen as good or bad, but rather as guidelines with which to explore the appropriateness of particular approaches to care in different contexts, critically and creatively. It is suggested that this is what was intended and, hopefully, achieved here.

Management aspects

Management features prominently in Orem's vocabulary. As already noted, the planning of nursing systems is seen as a management operation, and the production of self-care action is the self-care agency's equivalent managerial role. In reality, these two aspects of achieving self-medication are difficult to separate, and aspects of management are more easily considered in terms of the personnel involved in the exercise.

For the self-care agent (here, patient plus sister) factors which needed consideration included sufficient time for teaching input, methods of reinforcement and feedback and optimising time for discharge. In practice, teaching tended to centre on drug administration times (except for the initial session), both through convenience and relevance. This had implications for reinforcement (verbal), since it more accurately related to patient behaviour where the whole of the self-care operation was carried out. Discharge timing depended on a mutual agreement that an optimum, and safe, level of care had been achieved.

With regard to nursing colleagues, activity centred on discussion and teaching based on the self-care and rehabilitation ethos. It was here, perhaps, that the co-ordinator could more rigorously have applied a strategy based on learning theory. The failure to integrate the cognitive, affective and behavioural components of the individual nurse's approach to the model led to the problem with inconsistency noted above.

Other members of the health team needed to be involved in Miss Jones' care, either for advice, support, parallel input or, again, consistency in approach. It was here the care planner needed to exercise the skills of co-ordination and communication towards the production of a unified course of action. This included liaison with doctors, occupational and physiotherapists, specialist advisers and, principally, the ward pharmacist. The latter helped to devise the 'counselling' programme and formed a backup to nursing resources in the shape of knowledge, experience, patient teaching skills and, importantly, encouragement.

Of course, no nursing enterprise can succeed without the initial authority to proceed. Permission is needed from nursing management for self-medication where its principles extend beyond present policy. Where they do, skills of diplomacy and of creative thinking may be called for to circumvent apparent obstacles and achieve a modus vivendi where self-care principles can be maximised. It is to the credit of Orem's model that it can be successfully adapted to operate within such constraints.

Conclusion

This discussion has attempted to look at one particular nursing problem as it related to one particular individual, and at how the application of a comprehensive theory of nursing influenced problem-solving measures and outcomes. The nursing care which Miss Jones received may not have been ideal but neither, on the other hand, were its aims over-idealistic; the use of Orem's nursing model helped to provide a realistic course of action, to highlight strengths and weaknesses of nursing care and to provide a reference point from which future care-planning could develop.

References

Aggleton P & Chalmers H 1985 Orem's self-care model. *Nursing Times*, 81, 1: 36–39.

American Society of Hospital Pharmacists 1978 *Medication teaching manual: a guide for patient counselling.*

Anna DJ, Christensen DG, Hohon SA *et al.* 1978 Implementing Orem's conceptual framework. *Journal of Nursing Administration*, 8, 11: 8–11.

Atkinson L, Gibson IJM & Andrews J 1977 The difficulties of old people taking drugs. *Age and Ageing*, 6, 1: 44.

Atkinson L, Gibson IJM & Andrews J 1978 An investigation into the ability of elderly patients continuing to take prescribed drugs after discharge. *Gerontology*, 24: 225–34.

Baxendale C, Gourlay M & Gibson IJM 1978 A self-medication re-training programme. *British Medical Journal*, 2: 1278–9.

Barofsky I 1977 (Ed) *Medication compliance: a behavioural management approach.* Charles B. Slack Inc., New Jersey.

Becker MH, Maiman LA, Kirscht JP *et al.* 1979 Patient perceptions and compliance: recent studies of the Health Belief Model. In: Haynes *et al.*, see below.

Bromley DB 1974 *The psychology of human ageing.* 2nd Ed. Penguin, Harmondsworth.

Butterfield SE 1983 In search of commonalities: an analysis of two theoretical frameworks. *International Journal of Nursing Studies*, 20, 1: 15–22.

Campbell C 1984 Orem's story. *Nursing Mirror*, 159, 13: 28–30.

Christopher LJ, Ballinger BR, Shepherd, AMM *et al.* 1978 Drug prescribing patterns in the elderly: a cross-sectional study of in-patients. *Age and Ageing*, 7: 74.

Crome P, Akehurst M & Keet J 1980 Drug compliance in elderly hospital in-patients. *The Practitioner*, 224: 782–5.

Dall CE & Gresham L 1982 Promoting effective drug-taking behaviour in the elderly. *Nursing Clinics of North America*, 17, 2.

Davidson JR 1974 A trial of self-medication in the elderly. *Nursing Times*, 70, 3: 391–2.

Given BA & Given CW 1984 Creating a climate for compliance. *Cancer Nursing*, 7, 2: 139–47.

Harper DC 1984 Application of Orem's theoretical constructs to self-care medication behaviour in the elderly. *Advances in Nursing Science*, 6, 3: 29–44.

Hatch AM & Tapley A 1982 A self-administration system for elderly patients at Highbury Hospital. *Nursing Times*, 78, 42: 1773–4.

Haynes RB 1976 An initial review of the determinants of patient compliance with therapeutic regimens. In: Sackett, D. L. & Haynes, R. B. (Eds) *Compliance with therapeutic regimens.* Johns Hopkins University Press, Baltimore.

Haynes RB, Taylor DW & Sackett DL 1979 *Compliance in health care.* Johns Hopkins University Press, Baltimore.

Hogue CC 1979 Nursing and compliance. In: Haynes, R. B. Ibid.

Hulka BS 1979 Patient-clinician interaction and compliance. In: Haynes *et al*, see above.

Iveson-Iveson J 1982 Putting ideas into action. *Nursing Mirror*, 155, 16: 49

Joseph LS 1980 Self-care and the nursing process. *Nursing Clinics of North America*, 15, 1.

Kent G & Dalgleish M 1983 *Psychology and medical care.* Van Nostrand, Wokingham.

Kiernan PJ & Isaacs JB 1981 Use of drugs by the elderly. *Journal of the Royal Society of Medicine*, 74: 196–200.

Knust S & Quarn JM 1983 Integration of self-care theory with rehabilitation nursing. *Rehabilitation Nursing*, 8, 4: 26–28.

Law R & Chalmers C 1976 Medicines and elderly people: a general practice survey. *British Medical Journal*, 1: 565–8.

Lundin DV, Eros PA, Melloh J & Sands JE 1980 Education of independent elderly in the responsible use of prescription medication. *Drug Intelligence and Clinical Pharmacy*, 14: 335–42.

Macdonald ET, Macdonald JB & Phoenix M 1977 Improving drug compliance after hospital discharge. *British Medical Journal*, 2: 618–21.

Macdonald ET & Macdonald JB 1982 *Drug treatment in the elderly.* Wiley, Chichester.

Moughton M 1982 The patient: a partner in the health care process. *Nursing Clinics of North America*, 17, 3.

Norton JC 1982 *Introduction to medical psychology.* The Free Press, New York.

O'Hanrahan M & O'Malley K 1981 Compliance with drug treatment. *British Medical Journal*, 283: 298.

Orem DE 1980 *Nursing: concepts of practice.* 2nd Ed. McGraw-Hill, New York.

Parkin DM, Henney CR, Quirk J & Crooks SJ 1976 Deviation from prescribed treatment after discharge from hospital. *British Medical Journal*, 2: 686–8.

Potter M 1981 Medication compliance—a factor in the drug wastage problem. *Nursing Times* Occasional Paper, 77, 5: 17–20.

Qureshi KN & Hodkinson HM 1974 Evaluation of a ten question mental test in institutionalised elderly. *Age and Ageing*, 3: 152–57.

Reutter L 1984 Family health assessment—an integrated approach. *Journal of Advanced Nursing*, 9: 391–9.

Roberts R 1978 Self-medication trial for the elderly. *Nursing Times*, 74, 23: 976–7.

Roethlisberger F & Dickson E 1939 *Management and the worker.* Harvard University Press, Mass.

Roper N 1976 A model for nursing and nursology. *Journal of Advanced Nursing*, 1: 219–227.

Rosenberg SG 1976 Patient education: an educator's view. In: Sackett, D. L. & Haynes, R. B. (Eds) *Compliance with therapeutic regimens.* Johns Hopkins University Press, Baltimore.

Roy C 1980 The Roy adaptation model. In: Riehl, J. P. & Roy, C. (Eds) *Conceptual models for nursing practice.*

Appleton-Century-Crofts, Norwalk.

Royal College of Physicians 1984 Medication for the elderly. *Journal of the Royal College of Physicians*, **18**: 1.

Shannon M 1983 Self-medication in the elderly. *Nursing Mirror*, **157**, 15: Clinical Forum, 9.

Smith DL 1977 *Medication guide for patient counselling.* Lea & Febiger, Philadelphia.

Smith P & Andrews J 1983 Drug compliance not so bad, knowledge not so good—the elderly after hospital discharge. *Age and Ageing*, **12**, 4: 336–42.

Swift CG 1982 Practical management of drug therapy in the elderly. In: *Demonstration centres in rehabilitation newsletter*, January. Kingston General, Hull.

Wandless I & Davie JW 1977 Can drug compliance in the elderly be improved? *British Medical Journal*, **1**: 379–81.

Weibert RT & Deen DA 1980 *Improving patient medication compliance.* Medical Economics Co., New Jersey.

Williamson J 1978 Prescribing problems in the elderly. *British Medical Journal*, **220**: 749–55.

WHO 1946 *Constitution of the World Health Organization.* WHO, New York.

Appendix I

PATIENT PROFILE

PERSONAL DETAILS

Name   Emily Jones

Address   1, High Street, Newtown

Tel. No.   123-4567

Next of kin details   Agnes Jones, sister, 85 yrs   S/A

Occupation/interests   Watching T.V.

Access details   Entryphone

G.P. details   Dr Smith, High Street Surgery

Sex   F

Age/d.o.b.   87 yrs

Marital status   S

Religion   C/E

SOCIAL DETAILS

Environmental

Housing   Ground floor sheltered housing. Warden Mr Brown 123-7654

Sick room   Central heating. Good facilities

Washing/toilet facilities   Easy access, but no aids

Supporting services   Home help weekly. Luncheon club

Interpersonal

Composition of household   Patient and sister

Family structure:

   communication   Sometimes limited by pt's mild cognitive impairment

   role relationship   Both previously independent providers. Little overt interaction

   power structure   Neither very assertive. "Laissez-faire" tendency

   value systems   Both respect independence and privacy

Family perception of health situation

   Emily aware of breathing difficulties and effect on overall ability. Agnes little involved & tends to overlook problems, though supports sister.

MEDICAL DETAILS

Previous relevant medical history

   Rheumatic fever (as child); arthritis; variable shortness of breath for years.

History of present condition

   Increasing breathlessness and cough due to not taking diuretics. Occasional urinary incontinence and decreasing mobility.

Diagnoses

   Left ventricular failure; chronic obstructive airways disease.

Drug regimen

   Phyllocontin 225 mg b.d. Prednisone 30 mg o.d. Frusemide 40 mg b.d. Amiloride 5 mg o.d. Cetiprin 200 mg nocté.

Appendix II

NURSING ASSESSMENT

SELF-CARE REQUISITES	SELF-CARE DEMANDS	SELF-CARE ABILITY TO MEET DEMANDS i) **knowledge** ii) **motivation** iii) **skills**
Universal Provision of care associated with elimination processes and excrements	Pattern of elimination: Ability to walk to toilet 2–3 hourly. Ability to carry out mechanical functions without discomfort or difficulty. Care practices: Able to deal with clothing. Maintenance of body hygiene. Environment remains clean.	i) Sometimes forgets to go to toilet and wash herself. ii) Reliant on others to prompt. Sister not always involved. iii) Arthritis limits: —ability to get to toilet in time —ability to deal with clothing —ability to micturate in appropriate place.
Promotion of normal functioning	Awareness of effects of incontinence and decreased activity on personal independence and dignity. Adaptation of activities and relationships to preserve same.	i) Lacks insight into effects of physical limits on overall functioning though appreciates concept of dignity. ii) Therefore little remedial motivation in this sphere. iii) Cognitive/motor skill connection lacking.
Life-span/age-related (developmental) Increase in learning power to cope with drug schedule	Instruction in drug purpose and drug taking. Remember what to take, how and when. Behavioural change to effect compliance.	i) Does not know what drugs she is taking. ii) Wants to get better and take own pills. iii) Can open pill bottle when prompted, remove pill and replace lid.

Appendix II   NURSING ASSESSMENT (continued)

SELF-CARE REQUISITES	SELF-CARE DEMANDS	SELF-CARE ABILITY TO MEET DEMANDS i) knowledge ii) motivation iii) skills
Health-deviation Carry out prescribed measures directed at managing breathing difficulties and residual effects	Willing to participate in investigative and monitoring measures. Able to take drugs independently as prescribed. Adapt activity to limits that will not incapacitate breathing. Adopt position maximising inspiratory capacity.	i) Not aware of nature of disease or management. ii) Wants to breathe more easily but does not initiate action (i.e ask for help/advice). iii) Cannot take drugs independently. Has not found optimum exercise level. Has learned to sit upright.

Appendix III

NURSING CARE PLAN

SELF-CARE DEFICIT	OBJECTIVE	NURSING SYSTEM—METHOD OF ASSISTANCE i) wholly compensatory ii) partly compensatory iii) supportive/educative	RATIONALE
① Breathing Lacks understanding of disorder	Understands illness	iii) Explain simply why breathing difficult.	Baseline for self-care activity.
Lacks ability to take drugs independently	Takes drugs independently when condition permits	ii) Administer drugs until symptoms abate then as for problem ②.	
Lacks ability to gauge optimum exercise level for condition	Calculates, and engages in, correct exercise level for condition	i) ii) iii) Assist walking. Notice when breathless. Encourage independent mobility to this level.	Will retain independent mobility and realise association between movement and breathing.
Lacks motivation to engage in self-care	Expresses and demonstrates desire for self-care	ii) iii) Assist then withdraw support in self-care activities. Reward achievements with praise.	Will gain confidence and associate self-care behaviour with reward. Self-care is learned behaviour.
② Drugs Lacks knowledge and understanding of drug schedule.	Able to explain what drugs due when	iii) Explain, and reinforce over time, nature and purpose of drug regime.	Learning = knowledge + understanding + practice
Lacks ability to take drugs independently due to above.	Able to take drugs according to prescription independently before discharge	iii) Allow opportunity to discuss, select and administer own drugs at each round. Give positive feedback if operation carried out correctly.	
③ Elimination Forgets to go to toilet and to wash (relies on reminders).	Remembers/reminded to go to toilet and wash	iii) Remind to go to toilet 2 hourly.	Behaviour modification→ self-care.
Difficulty in walking to toilet, dealing with clothes and positioning on toilet.	Able to walk to toilet, sit on toilet and manage clothes without undue distress	i) Liaise with physio and occ. therapist for assessment/provision of: —zimmer/stick —raised toilet seat —altered clothing.	Limitation of painful movement to arthritic joints → greater independence.
Some nocturnal incontinence	Incontinence contained/controlled	iii) Explain purpose of anti-cholinergic drug added to regime. Discuss with pt. possibility of 'high' commode.	Understanding → acceptance/ compliance + control over medication.

3

A study in adaptation: care for an elderly incontinent man, based on Roy's Adaptation model

Alan Pearson

Introduction

Urinary incontinence is an increasing problem in Western societies and is often faced by elderly people as the ageing process develops (Brink 1980). Although virtually all members of the multidisciplinary team have some expertise to contribute towards resolving the problem, it is usually dependent upon the input of professional nurses, both at home and in hospital. Thorough assessment, realistic goal setting, clear care planning and ongoing, careful evaluation can all lead to either the restoration of continence or the development of strategies to overcome the impairment to independent living which it causes (Dufautt 1978).

Direction is given to the nursing process in this area of major concern by the use of an organising framework, or conceptual model. As the ultimate goal in such cases is adaptation of the whole person, a model based on this concept is thought by many to be useful.

Adaptation as a concept in nursing

The concept of adaptation assumes that people are open systems which respond to stimuli from both inside and outside the person. The responses to such stimuli are termed adaptation. In its truest sense, it is neither positive or negative—it is simply a response to any internal or external stimuli. In its application today, however, adaptation is seen as a positive response, whilst a negative response is termed maladaptation. Adaptation leads to homeostasis or integrity in the physiological, social and psychological sense. Physiological adaptation is stability of the internal environment of the person; psychological adaptation is the possession of self esteem and identity, and social adaptation is the meeting of expectations in the society in which the person lives. Illness and disease—that is, a patho-physiological state—are physiological maladaptations, whilst some mental illness and anti-social or deviant behaviour are examples of maladaptation in the psychological and social realms, respectively.

Thus, the individual is viewed holistically, and nursing is charged with a concern for the physical and psychosocial needs of those who receive its service.

The Roy Adaptation Model for Nursing (Roy 1974)

This model focuses on the individual as a system, made up of sub-systems and living in a supra-system. Roy views the person as a bio-psycho-social creature, who must be considered as a unified whole. The goal of nursing is to promote an individual's adaptation to internal and external changes. People must respond or adapt to any changes that occur using innate and acquired mechanisms, in order to maintain homeostasis or integrity.

The changes, or *stimuli*, which necessitate adaptation impinge on the person and create unusual demands. Three types of stimuli are described:

1 *Focal stimuli*: These are changes or situations which immediately affect the individual, such as a broken limb, the loss of a loved one or a pain in a specific site.
2 *Contextual stimuli*: These are all the other stimuli present which may influence a response to the focal stimulus, such as anaemia, poor housing or other surrounding circumstances.
3 *Residual stimuli*: These are the characteristics, values and attitudes of the individual which have developed from past experience. For example, a person's background may lead him to accept the death of a spouse easily, whilst another may find this difficult to do. The individual who has suffered much pain in the past may well be able to cope with post-operative pain, whilst it may be extremely difficult to bear for someone who has never experienced severe pain before.

Responses to such stimuli occur within an individual's *adaptation zone*. This zone is the area in which the individual can adapt in a positive way. Provided that all the stimuli bombarding the person fall within the zone, he will be able to maintain integrity and responses will be positive or *adaptive*. If the stimuli are too great and

therefore move outside the person's own zone, the responses made will not result in integrity and will be negative, or *maladaptive*. Thus, this personal adaptation zone is specific to each individual.

For example, when facing a huge overdraft at the bank, one individual may arrange to see the bank manager, discuss a possible loan from a friend and investigate the possibility of selling something to help with the financial crisis—a positive adaptation within this person's own zone. Another, however, may withdraw from others, worry about the situation and consider ending it all—a negative adaptation because the stimuli extended outside the person's own adaptation zone.

Roy suggests that human needs can be divided into four types, and integrity of the person revolves around the meeting of these needs. She terms them the four modes of adaptation.

Physiological Mode: This is associated with the structure and function of the body. Six basic needs are identified, which must be met to achieve integrity:

1 Exercise and rest
2 Nutrition
3 Elimination
4 Fluid and electrolytes
5 Oxygenation and circulation
6 Regulation of temperature, senses and endocrines

Self Concept: This is how the person perceives himself and two distinct areas can be distinguished. The physical self is related to the person's mental perception of himself and is directed by feelings, sensations, appearance and body image. The personal self relates to the individual's own standards, beliefs, morals and behaviours. Rambo (1984) says that self concept 'consists of feelings and beliefs that permit an individual to know who he or she is and feel that self is adequate in meeting needs and desires'.

Role function: This is psychosocial integrity of the individual in assuming those roles which have to be adopted in his life and in meeting the

Fig. 3.1   Stimuli which necessitate adaptation

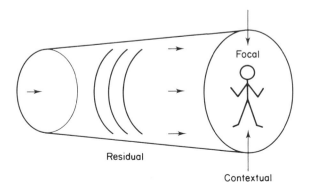

expectations of society of those roles. Roy describes role as 'the title given to the individual—mother, son, student, carpenter—as well as the behaviours that society expects a person to perform in order to maintain the title'. Rambo (1984) suggests that most people have primary, secondary and tertiary roles. Primary roles are relatively definite and are predetermined, for example girl, woman, boy and man. Secondary roles are relatively permanent but may be chosen, such as parent, nurse, student, wife or husband. Tertiary roles are usually temporary and freely chosen, such as committee member, scout leader or church organist.

Interdependence: This is the balance between dependence and independence. Dependence is a need to rely on others for care, support and approval. Independence is the ability to decide upon, and initiate, successful actions. Interdependence is the balance between these two extremes, where the individual can function alone, without rejecting a sharing with others in daily living.

Elhart *et al.* (1978) describe how the adaptation process can be related to the nursing process:

Assessment
First level
assessment—recognising the patient's positive and negative behaviours in each of the four adaptive modes.
Second level
assessment—identifying factors influencing behaviour and classifying them as focal, contextual and residual stimuli.

Planning
Selecting appropriate intervention, which may involve:
　　Reducing or limiting stress (stimuli outside zone)
　　Preventing additional stress
　　Supporting adaptations
　　Limiting adaptations
　　Altering adaptations
　　Interrupting adaptations
　　Supplementing adaptations

Implementing
Carrying out the selected intervention.

Evaluation
Reassessing behaviours in the four adaptive modes to determine satisfactory resolution of the problem or need for reassessment.

First level assessment involves observing behaviour in the four modes and detecting areas of concern. Second level assessment concentrates on those areas of concern and determining the focal, contextual or residual stimuli leading to each behaviour. Problems are therefore identified and goals are established in terms of behavioural outcomes. The nursing interventions selected aim at removing the focal stimuli or changing the contextual or residual stimuli, that is, removing the cause or broadening the adaptation zone.

The problem of incontinence of urine

Urinary incontinence is the inability to control the passing of urine, which may be either temporary, prolonged or permanent according to the causes and contributing factors associated with the individual. The crucial determinant in controlling urination is control of the bladder sphincter, which requires normal voluntary and involuntary muscle action co-ordinated by a normal urethrobladder reflex (Brink 1980).

Urine passes from the kidneys to the bladder along the ureters and is propelled by peristaltic contractions of the smooth muscle in the ureter walls. The bladder itself has walls of thick layers of smooth muscle and contraction of the walls increases the pressure of urine inside the bladder. When the bladder is relaxed, the internal urethral sphincter is closed, but contraction of the bladder pulls open the sphincter. The external urethral sphincter is a circular layer of skeletal muscle which surrounds the urethra below the base of the bladder. When contracted, it can hold the urethra closed against very strong contractions of the bladder (Vander *et al.* 1975).

Passing urine occurs through a local spinal reflex which can be influenced by higher brain centres. Bladder contraction occurs through the stimulation of the parasympathetic nerves supplying the bladder muscle. Such contractions automatically open the internal urethral sphincter. The bladder wall also contains 'stretch receptors' which, when excited, transmit nerve impulses into the spinal cord leading to a conscious desire to pass urine and a subconscious reflex called the 'micturition reflex'. The reflex signal is transmitted to the bladder wall which contracts and relaxes the internal urethral sphincter. Urine cannot be passed, however, until the external urethral sphincter relaxes. In the healthy adult, the reflex can be resisted by the individual consciously keeping the external sphincter closed. When it is appropriate to pass urine, the individual can do so because the conscious portion of the brain will relax the external sphincter by inhibiting the normal impulses being sent to it through the pudic nerve. When an individual resists the urge to pass urine, the reflex usually subsides and remains inhibited for up to an hour before it returns again. As the bladder becomes more and more filled, however, the desire to pass urine becomes stronger. Babies automatically pass urine every time the bladder fills because they have not developed voluntary control over the external urethral sphincter (Guyton 1974).

The causes of urinary incontinence

The uncontrolled passing of urine may arise because of a disturbance in the individual's consciousness, in the micturition reflex or in the patency of the external urethral sphincter. In the elderly, the degeneration of intellectual capacity, as in dementia or following a cerebrovascular accident, is a major cause of incontinence. The weakening of muscular efficiency in general also affects the patency of the external urethral sphincter in the process of ageing.

Long and Phipps (1985) list the following major causes of incontinence:

Cause of urinary incontinence	Awareness of need to void	Cortical ability to inhibit voiding	Reflex arc	Bladder response to filling	Result
Cerebral clouding	Impaired	Impaired	Intact	Normal	Uncontrolled voiding because of reflex response
Infection	Intact	Intact, but overcome by strong reflex response	Abnormally stimulated	Heightened	Voiding because of strong reflex response (urgency)
Disturbance of CNS pathways (cortical lesions)	Diminished	Impaired	Intact	Heightened	Voiding because of reflex response
Disturbance of urethrobladder reflex. Upper motor neurone lesion	Destroyed	Destroyed	Intact but deranged	Heightened	Voiding because of reflex response.
Lower motor neurone lesion	Destroyed	Destroyed	Destroyed or impaired	Diminished to absent	Distention or incomplete emptying
Tissue damage	Intact	Intact, but not functional because of poor muscle response	Intact	Normal	Loss of control of voiding because of muscular impairment

Elhart *et al.* (1978) describe incontinence as ' . . . one of the most devastating of physical problems from the patient's viewpoint, and it causes much embarrassment and emotional disturbance. It is a common problem for many geriatric patients who have suffered a cerebrovascular accident or those with atonic muscles'. The literature in general emphasises the enormity of the problem amongst the elderly (Shephard *et al.* 1982), the need for skilled specialist nursing (Blannin 1983) and the qualitative benefits of systematic assessment and intervention on the lives of elderly people suffering from incontinence (Wells 1980, Portnoi 1981, Lowthian 1977).

Adaptation and incontinence

The concept of adaptation to help patients who are incontinent has much to offer. It focuses on the whole person and demands detailed analysis of the stimuli which are impinging on the individual and leading to the problem. Incontinence is a physiological phenomenon, which is fundamentally related to the individual's concept of self, role function and interdependence. Roy's model focuses on the individual as a composite of inter-related systems, where it is impossible to separate the physical aspects of incontinence from the psychological and social aspects of the person.

Although nursing intervention is determined both by the specific type and cause of incontinence, and the individual's own circumstances, the nursing process itself can be generally applied from Roy's perspective.

Mr. Peter Moss was referred to his local community hospital by the attending District Nursing Sister for assessment and rehabilitation. Mr. Moss's major problem was incontinence, and applying the concept of adaptation to his nursing care explains the use of Roy's model in practice.

A study in patient care

Mr. Moss lives with his 60 year old daughter in a rented local authority house in the rural village of High Ridge. He is 81 years old, has suffered from Parkinsons disease for 9 years and has lived with his daughter for 15 years since the death of his wife. The District Nurse has been visiting for $2\frac{1}{2}$ years to help Mr. Moss into the bath and, over the last two years, to support the daughter because of her father's increasing incontinence. An examination by a urologist $1\frac{1}{2}$ years ago concluded that little could be done about the incontinence and the general practitioner was advised to help Mr. Moss and his daughter to establish a toileting programme and to explore various aids to continence. The only aids eventually found to be acceptable were 'Kanga' pants and pads, and a commode. Over the last few months, the daughter has become increasingly distressed about caring for her father and notable tension in the house has been observed by the District Nurse. She has requested an admission to the community hospital, supported by the GP, to:

a) give Mr. Moss, his daughter and the District Nurse a break
b) assess the incontinence and develop strategies to cope with it.

The referral was accepted and Mr. Moss was admitted two weeks later. On admission, he was allocated a primary nurse, who began to assess him and identify problems. The initial assessment took place over the day of admission and was recorded on an assessment sheet based on Roy's model (Fig. 3.2).

As well as collecting basic biographical information, Mr. Moss's behaviour in the four adaptive modes, and the associated stimuli, were observed and recorded (first level assessment). Using this data, the nurse and patient were able to identify a number of problems (second level assessment). The major problems relating to incontinence were:

1 Unable to control passing urine
2 Finds it difficult to accept increased dependence
3 Feels guilty about the extra work he creates for his daughter
4 Has never adjusted to his loss of role as husband and father
5 Feels unable to ask his daughter for help.

Specific behavioural goals related to each of these problems were agreed upon between the nurse and patient and nursing action to achieve them was prescribed. This formed the plan of care for Mr. Moss (Fig 3.3).

The plan of care and the resulting nursing action focuses on the patient's problem of incontinence in the four adaptive modes, and not just the physical phenomena. The nursing care focuses on the stimuli which lead to the behaviours observed and the overall goal is to either remove or control the stimuli, or to promote adaptation.

Problem 1 Inability to control passing urine

Previous investigation of Mr. Moss suggested that little could be done to help total alleviation of the problem. Nursing intervention therefore involved an attempt to keep the bladder empty to avoid uncontrollable voiding. Over the course of three days, the habit training chart showed that regular toileting reduced bedwetting to one episode per night (Fig. 3.4). The use of a Kylie sheet meant that Mr. Moss remained relatively

Fig. 3.2 Patient assessment sheet

| Surname: MOSS | Forenames: PETER JOHN | D.O.B. 1/11/1904 | Age 81 | Sex M | MSW |
| | | | | | REL |

Address: 18, MILLFIELD LANE HIGH RIDGE.	Telephone: High Ridge 621	N.O.K. Daughter (Muriel Moss)	Address: S/A	Telephone:

Meaningful Others:
Married son in New Zealand (George Moss)—have not met for 12 years—send Christmas cards to each other only.

Prefers to be addressed as:
MR. MOSS

Reason for admission:
Referred by Carol Evans (District Nursing Sister) to give daughter a rest and to assess incontinence.

Relevant medical information:
Parkinson's disease since 1977

Occupation:
Retired agricultural labourer

Usual daily living pattern:
Up at 9 am—toast for breakfast. Lunch (sandwich) at 1 pm then sleep in chair in afternoon. Meat & veg. for dinner at 6 pm. Watches TV in evening. Bed at 9–10 pm. Walks with Zimmer.

Baseline data (Urine/TPR/BP etc):
Urine—N.A.D.   T 36.8   P 84   R 20   B.P. $\frac{150}{90}$

Primary Nurse: Steve Wilson	**Doctor:** Roger Potter

Fig. 3.2 (continued)

ASSESSMENT

FIRST LEVEL   *SECOND LEVEL*

Behaviour:	Stimulus		
	Focal	Contextual	Residual
Physiological: **Elimination** Incontinent of urine about twice during night. Dry in mornings, but often wet in afternoon when sleeping on settee.	Loss of bladder control	Aged 81 years Parkinson's disease Difficulty in transfer-ring from bed to chair	
Self Concept 1. Badly misses being able to look after himself. 2. Feels very guilty about creating extra work for daughter; consequently, can't talk to her about it.	Restricted mobility Poor memory Has never perceived daughter as indepen-dent adult.	Socially isolated Circumstances have forced daughter to be his most frequent companion.	Has always seen him-self as head of household
Role function Feels that incontinence denies him the possibility of behaving as a responsible adult.	He no longer has con-trol over the household	Now lives in daughter's home	Sees incontinence as childish behaviour which is inappropriate for a mature adult
Interdependence Says he has never liked other people doing things for him and has always managed his own life.	Physical condition necessitates a need for some help from daughter.		Brought up to stand on own feet.

comfortable despite the incontinence and his skin remained intact. However, the afternoon inconti-nence persisted. The care plan was altered to include an extra toileting at 1.30 pm, but this still had no effect. Mr. Moss was reluctant to forfeit his afternoon 'nap' when it was suggested that he should be woken soon after he began to sleep, and the use of an incontinence appliance incorporat-ing a sheath was not acceptable to him. Mr. Moss suggested that extra pads should be used after the 1.30 toileting, so that the chair remained dry. This strategy was successful, and thus an adap-tation to the focal stimulus was made and the behaviour in the physiological mode was modified.

Problem 2 Difficulty in accepting increased dependence

The nursing intervention related to information-giving encouraged Mr. Moss to discuss this difficulty, but he was unable to come to terms with it or to change the behaviour of failing to talk

Fig. 3.3 Care plan

Problem	Goal	Nursing Intervention
1. Unable to control passing urine.	1. Will remain dry all day. 2. Will not be wet more than once during night. 3. Skin will remain intact. 4. Will be odour free.	1. Help to use commode at following times: 9am, 12md, 3pm, 6pm, 9pm, 12mn. 2. Record habit training chart at above times. 3. Help to apply zinc cream to sacrum at 9am, 12md, 6pm and 11pm 4. Wear Kanga pants and pads whilst up. 5. Kylie sheet in bed at night.
2. Finds it difficult to accept reduced ability to be independent.	Will say that this difficulty feels less to him.	1. Discuss the nature of dependence when appropriate. 2. Give Age Concern/Disabled Living Foundation publication to read. 3. Encourage him to express feelings when appropriate.
3. Feels guilty about the extra work he creates for his daughter.	1. Work load for daughter will be less than it is now. 2. Will indicate that he has less feelings of guilt.	1. Discuss situation, and goal, with daughter and Mr. Moss together. 2. Arrange laundry service.
4. Has never adjusted to his loss of role as husband and father.	Will discuss his feelings openly.	Bring up subject at least daily and offer opportunity to listen.
5. Feels unable to ask his daughter for help.	Will provide daughter with a list of specific helping acts.	1. Discuss daily living needs. 2. Identify all of these which require assistance. 3. Compile definitive list of help needed by daughter. 4. Arrange meeting with Mr. Moss, daughter, District Nurse and Community O. T. to discuss list.

to his daughter. The problem was, however, to be pursued after discharge by the District Nurse.

Problem 3 Feelings of guilt about the extra work created for daughter

The reduction of workload for the daughter lessened the causes of guilt and the open discussion between her and Mr. Moss led to a greater closeness and acknowledgement of guilt feelings. As in problem 2, Mr. Moss's self concept of an independent adult subjected to unwanted dependence remained strong, and a lessening of the stress which lead to guilt feelings was seen as more appropriate than trying to revise his own concept of self.

Fig. 3.4 Habit retraining chart

Name of Patient __Mr. Moss__   PRIMARY NURSE __Steve Wilson__

Habit Retraining Chart

Help to Commode at
9am, 12md, 3pm, 6pm, 9pm, 12mn. (+1.30pm)

Date	DAY 8 9 10 11 12 1 2 3 4 5 6 7 8 9	MANAGEMENT	NIGHT 10 11 12 1 2 3 4 5 6 7	MANAGEMENT
1	□ O Δ Δ		□ O O	
2	Δ Δ O □ Δ		Δ O	
3	□ Δ O □ Δ Δ		Δ O	
4	Δ Δ □□O □ Δ Δ	extra toilet at 1.30pm.	Δ	
5	Δ □ OΔ Δ □ Δ		Δ	
6	Δ Δ ΔO □ Δ Δ		Δ O	
7	Δ Δ □ Δ O Δ □		Δ O	
8	Δ □ □O Δ □ Δ		Δ	
9	Δ Δ Δ □ O □ Δ		□ O	

KEY   State of Patient

Dry = X
Incontinent of Urine = O

Result of Toileting

Urine passed in toilet = Δ
Urine not passed in toilet = □
Refused or absent = ✳

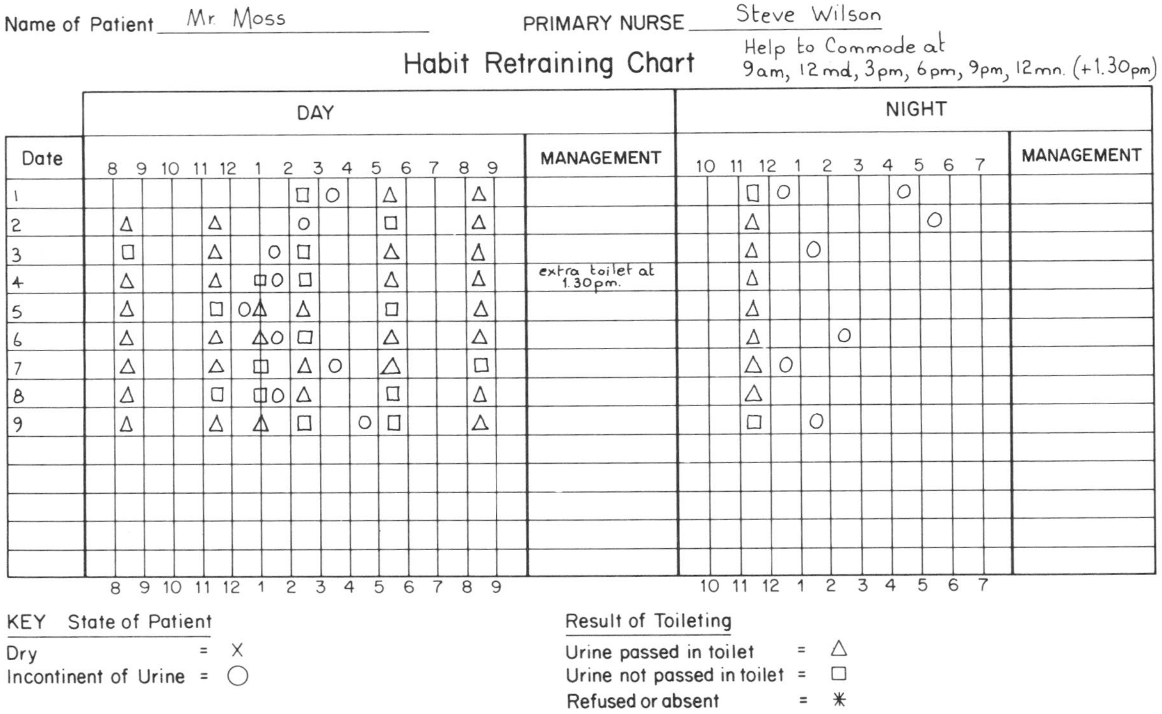

Problem 4 Has never adjusted to his loss of role as husband and father

Mr. Moss was able to discuss his feelings of loss about his wife and the embarrassment he felt at his daughter almost taking her place.

Problem 5 Feels unable to ask his daughter for help

The construction of a list of needs helped Mr. Moss to acknowledge what they were, and to face up to requesting help from his daughter. The daughter, too, was able to show her father that she was willing to give the assistance he needed and she, in turn, felt more able to request help from professional sources.

Mr. Moss was discharged home after 9 days in the community hospital, having achieved some positive adaptations of behaviour in the four adaptive modes, as discussed above.

Conclusion

The Roy Adaptation model emphasises helping people to adapt to stimuli and to modify maladaptive behaviour. It incorporates assessment of behaviour in the four adaptive modes of physiological functioning, self concept, role function and independence. Incontinence in the elderly always involves adaptation in all four modes, and the concept of adaptation therefore seems an appropriate framework for action in nursing incontinent people. The process of living is, perhaps, nothing more than the process of adaptation to internal and external stimuli, and the process of nursing anyone is the promotion of adaptation.

The advantages and disadvantages of Roy's model

As this study of care demonstrates, Roy's concepts can be used creatively to help those with incontinence and presumably, other problems associated with ageing. Adaptation is a relevant overriding goal in care of the elderly and the four adaptive modes offer a useful framework for assessment and planning.

The model depends, however, on the acquisition of a new vocabulary. It is also very 'person' centred, and his or her family and meaningful others may be seen as aspects of the surrounding environment. Ageing often leads to a decline in physical functioning and some imagination is needed to focus on functional ability in the activities of daily living when adaptation is used as the primary concept.

The complexity of the model and its theoretical basis make it difficult to recommend its wider use in care of the elderly in the UK. Its underlying theories and propositions require much more rigorous testing before they can be uncritically accepted and their unfamiliarity to British nurses may lead to a rejection of model based practice, rather than an improvement in standards.

References

Blannin JP 1983 The role of the nursing continence advisor. *Physiotherapy*, 10:69, 4:111–112.

Brink C 1980 Urinary continence/incontinence. Assessing the problem. *Geriatric Nursing*, 1, 4: 241–245, 275.

Dufautt K 1978 Urinary incontinence: United States and British nursing perspectives. *Journal of Gerontological Nursing*, 4, 2: 28–33.

Elhart D, Firsich SC, Gragg SH & Rees OM 1978 *Scientific principles in nursing.* C. V. Mosby, St. Louis.

Guyton AC 1974 *Function of the human body.* 4th Ed. W. B. Saunders, Philadelphia.

Long BC & Phipps WJ 1985 *Essentials of medical-surgical nursing.* C. V. Mosby, St. Louis.

Lowthian P 1977 The elderly—a challenge to nursing—5. Frequent micturition and its significance. *Nursing Times*, 73, 46: 1809–1813.

Portnoi VA 1981 Urinary incontinence in the elderly. *American Family Physician*, 23, 6: 151–154.

Rambo BJ 1984 *Adaptation nursing: assessment and intervention.* W. B. Saunders, Philadelphia.

Roy C 1974 The Roy adaptation model. In: Riehl, J. P. & Roy, C. (Eds) *Conceptual models for nursing practice.* Appleton-Century-Crofts, Norwalk.

Shephard AM, Blannin JP & Fenely RC 1982 Changing attitudes in the management of urinary incontinence—the need for specialist nursing. *British Medical Journal (Clinical Research)*, 284, 6316: 645–646.

Vander AJ, Sherman JH & Luciano DS 1975 *Human physiology. The mechanisms of body function.* 2nd Ed. Tate McGraw-Hill, New Delhi.

Wells T 1980 Promoting urine control in older adults. Scope of the problem. *Geriatric Nursing*, 1, 4: 236–240, 275.

4

The depressed, elderly individual: an analysis of the use of Saxton and Hyland's Stress Adaptation model

Alan Skeath

In this chapter, some of the problems experienced by depressed elderly people will be examined. Within this context, it is also proposed to examine the usefulness of a particular model of nursing care; the stress adaptation model. However, before considering this model and what it has to offer, the problem of depression must be reviewed.

Depression can be defined as a deviation of mood from one that is normal for the individual to one that reflects a degree of psychomotor retardation. It may be accompanied by feelings of hopelessness and despair. Depression is thus not specifically defined as a disease or illness. It is a problem that, at some time or other, is experienced by each and every one of us. In its milder form, depression can be seen as a mood swing within the tolerance of acceptable limits and which invariably resolves itself rapidly, enabling the individual to return to his normal state of functioning. These bouts of mild depression can be precipitated by, for example, loss of a cheque book or the fact that the car, just back from the garage following a service, will not start. On other occasions, there are no ready explanations for feelings of moroseness, but the individual recognises that he feels unhappy.

How then does the depression which most people experience differ from the so-called 'clinical depression' which is usually regarded as one of the mental illnesses? There are a number of factors that could lead one to believe that an individual might be clinically depressed:

1 *The duration of the depression.* Any person who complains of symptoms of a depressive nature that have been present for a period of six months or more should be considered clinically depressed.

2 *The rationality of the explanations given to account for the depression.* The individual might suggest that a minor physical complaint is causing him or her to be depressed, the magnitude of the physical complaint being out of keeping with the degree of depression observed.

3 *The ability or otherwise of the person to explain how the problems of depression might be coped with and their preparedness or ability to take appropriate action.* It might be that the problems associated with the depression and indeed the depression itself could be alleviated if, for example, the individual were to change employment or marital status.

4 *Evidence of suicidal or homicidal tendencies.*

5 *The degree to which the problems interfere with the individual's daily life.* Do the problems prevent the person from getting up in the morning; do they interfere with the person's ability to relate to others; do they result in the individual using avoidance strategies such as not wanting to go to work?

Causes of depression in the elderly

The traditional approaches to the problems of mental illness and hence the identification of the causes and treatment of depression have been via a variety of medical models. The main areas of concern have centred upon the nature and cause of the illness, its diagnosis and cure. Different propositions have been put forward which have attempted to link depression with disturbances in biochemical function, particularly in respect to the lowering of transmitter substance levels in the central nervous system (Perry & Perry 1982). Other causative factors that have been suggested imply that the problem has either a socio-cultural basis (Kiev 1972) or a genetic origin (Cadoret *et al.* 1970). The possibility that depression is the result of an unmanageable level of stress that acts as a triggering mechanism has been postulated. Notwithstanding the very considerable amount of research that has gone into investigating the problems of depression, they still appear regularly.

It is certainly true that the use of physical agents, including both drugs and electroconvulsive therapy, might afford some short term relief when used in the treatment of certain selected patients. However, while not wishing to condemn the use of nor totally undermine the efficacy of physical methods of treatment, it must be stated that the observable evidence in terms of longlasting benefits is not encouraging. Witness the number of patients who are readmitted to hospital following initial treatment (Goble 1979, Pollit 1978). The revolving door phenomenon has frequently been observed and associated with the traditional institutional care of the depressed patient.

Szasz (1974) has stated that the problem of mental illness is essentially a psychological one and that to use a medical approach in attempting to alleviate it is quite inappropriate. Clare (1980) poses the question 'Does mental illness exist?' He suggests that what are commonly referred to as mental illnesses are in fact disordered interpersonal relationships. A sociological (Marxian) interpretation of mental illness is that it is a political tool of capitalist societies and can be used to exert power and social control. The dissenter, the handicapped or the elderly person who is unable to contribute to the economy is not tolerated within the society; he is debunked, degraded and subjected to incarceration because he is not productive in socio-economic terms.

Much of the foregoing suggests that the medical mode of approach to the problems of mental illness and hence depression is far from satisfactory and that alternative methods should be sought. Some indications as to the nature of possible alternative models are provided by the comments of Sarabin (1969) who questions the use of the term 'mental illness'. He prefers to refer to the problems categorised under this heading as being those of social dysfunctional conduct and suggests that treatment should be concerned with the transformation of social identities.

Depression is a universal phenomenon and Rowe (1985) has intimated that it is not an illness in terms of the physical sciences, but possibly an avoidance strategy which enables the individual to escape from the confrontations of unacceptable life or reality situations. This leads to the belief that depressed people have to be enabled to recognise their problems in their own terms and to devise appropriate alternative, more healthy, coping strategies. This enabling function is the most important aspect of the nurse's role. The nurse must be available to listen to, interpret and facilitate patients in the redefining or restructuring of their problems. Patients also need assistance in the examination and identification of more acceptable alternative solutions.

The incidence of depression in the elderly

This is not an easy statistic to identify accurately, mainly due to the difficulty of diagnosis. Many patients who are clinically depressed are also suffering from other psychiatric disorders and thus total numbers will depend on whether the depression has been diagnosed as a separate entity or not. Available figures indicate that, at any one time, some 4 per cent of the population over the age of 65 years suffer from depression (Godber 1978).

It is also known with a fair amount of certainty that the age groups in which the highest number of suicides occur is 75 years and over for men and

Fig. 4.1 Suicide rates by sex and age. Source: Office of Population Censuses and Surveys; General Register Office (Scotland); General Register Office (N. Ireland). (Social Trends 1985.)

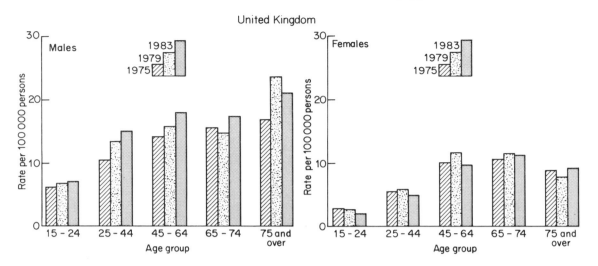

65–74 years for women (Fig. 4.1). If one assumes that, in many instances, depression is the root cause of suicide, then the nature and magnitude of the problem become clearer. It must be borne in mind, however, that not all suicides are the direct result of depression, and it is necessary to exercise caution when extrapolating from these figures. It might be interesting at this point to examine the possibility of taking suicide as the ultimate in avoidance techniques.

Precipitating factors

There are many factors that are likely to contribute to the onset of depression in the elderly. Some of the more common ones are:

Social isolation resulting from, for example: death of a spouse, children having moved away, physical handicap. The chances of having to live alone increase with age. Over the age of 65 years the problem is greater for women as they generally live longer than men. It can be seen from the following table that in 1983, 46.6 per cent of those aged 75 years or over and living in private households lived alone (56.8 per cent of all women and 28 per cent of men).

Table 4.1 Percentage of people in private households in each age group who live alone, 1973 and 1983. Source: General Household Survey, 1973 and 1983. (Social Trends 1985).

	Percentages	
	1973	1983
Percentage of people aged:		
16–24	0.5	0.9
25–44	2.4	4.2
45–64	8.1	9.3
65–74	25.7	27.6
75 or over	40.0	46.6
All aged 16 or over	6.7	8.7
Percentage of males aged:		
65–74	13.1	15.3
75 or over	24.2	28.4
Percentage of females aged:		
65–74	35.8	36.8
75 or over	48.0	56.8

Loss of income. From Fig. 4.2, it can be seen that 42 per cent of those with incomes at or below supplementary benefit level were single people over pensionable age. Approximately half of the

Fig. 4.2 Families with incomes at or below supplementary benefit level by family type, by tenure and by age of head (1981). Source: Dept of Health and Social Security, from Annual Statistical Enquiry and Family Expenditure Survey. (Social Trends 1985).

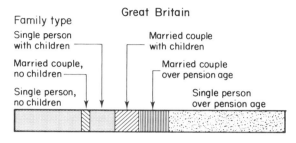

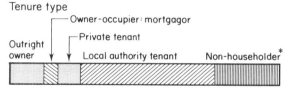

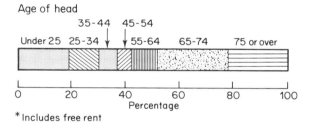

*Includes free rent

low income families were those in which the head of the family was aged 65 years or over.

Unsatisfactory housing. The English House Condition Surveys (1976 and 1981) indicated that, of the households that were headed by a retired person, 47 per cent lacked a bath; 33 per cent were unfit for accommodation; and 27 per cent were described as fit but in a serious state of disrepair.

Problems relating to social isolation, reduction in income and inadequate housing are precipitators of stress, which is frequently seen as a precursor of depression. Depression is possibly being employed as an avoidance strategy and used in order to escape from the more unacceptable problems of stress.

There are, of course, many other life events that give rise to stress and it is useful to study the impact they may have on the individual (Holmes & Holmes 1970). Death of a spouse (Greenblatt 1978, Richter 1984) has the greatest impact and it is worthwhile examining the extent to which bereavement can contribute to the problem of depression.

Table 4.2 Stress ratings of various life events. Adapted from Holmes, T. S. & Holmes, T. H. Short-term intrusions into life-style routine. *Journal of Psychosomatic Research*, 1970, 14, 121–132. Reprinted with permission of Pergamon Press, Ltd.

Events	Scale of Impact
Death of spouse	100
Divorce	73
Marital separation	65
Jail term	63
Death of close family member	63
Personal injury or illness	53
Marriage	50
Fired at work	47
Marital reconciliation	45
Retirement	45
Change in health of family member	44
Pregnancy	40
Sex difficulties	39
Gain of new family member	39
Business readjustment	39
Change in financial state	38
Death of close friend	37
Change to different line of work	36
Change in number of arguments with spouse	35
Mortgage over $10,000	31
Foreclosure of mortgage or loan	30
Change in responsibilities at work	29
Son or daughter leaving home	29
Trouble with in-laws	29
Outstanding personal achievement	28
Wife begins or stops work	26
Begin or end school	26
Change in living conditions	25
Revision of personal habits	24
Trouble with boss	23
Change in work hours or conditions	20
Change in residence	20

Table 4.2 (continued)

Events	Scale of Impact
Change in schools	20
Change in recreation	19
Change in church activities	19
Change in social activities	18
Mortgage or loan less than $10,000	17
Change in sleeping habits	16
Change in number of family get-togethers	15
Change in eating habits	15
Vacation	13
Christmas	12
Minor violations of the law	11

Bereavement is usually accompanied by a series of characteristic behaviours referred to collectively as the grief reaction. These behaviours represent a set sequence of emotional responses. The different phases are not always easy to identify separately and there may be some degree of overlapping. The duration of the phases is likely to vary from person to person. The following phases of the grief reaction are commonly described:

Anticipation
Anticipatory grief is that which is experienced after receiving the news that a close friend or relative is dying (Gerber *et al.* 1975). While having to cope with feelings of impending loss, the individual has to command sufficient strength and composure in order to comfort the dying person. This anticipatory period provides an opportunity for the individual to prepare for the impending death. It thus follows that, should death occur suddenly, there will be no anticipatory grieving. Failure to indulge in anticipatory grieving for whatever reason might lead to the experiencing of extreme forms of guilt and hence the manifestations of clinical depression.

Shock
It is usual for bereaved people to experience a period of shock during which they might find it difficult to express emotions. It is not uncommon during this stage for the individual to 'feel numb'. Other accompanying features include loss of appetite, agitation and insomnia. Intermittent grieving in terms of weeping and other expressions of sadness is likely to occur.

Anger
Sometimes the bereaved person expresses feelings of hostility (Stern *et al.* 1951). These may be directed towards those involved in caring for the dead person; towards the deceased, who may be blamed for not caring for himself; or towards other relatives. Occasionally the anger is directed against God, who is rebuked for having 'failed those who support Him'.

The expression of anger, while being useful in that it enables the individual to discharge feelings of emotion, can also exacerbate already existing tensions. It might serve ultimately to strain and sever family relationships at a time when support is most needed.

Control
A number of people, relatives, friends, clergymen and other close associates, are usually available to support the mourner following the death. They will help to make the individual feel that help is close at hand should it be required. They will provide a source of encouragement, enabling the mourner to express feelings and assisting in making the arrangements for the funeral. The mourner will usually react in an appreciative manner accepting the help and goodwill of all concerned in a dignified and controlled way.

Denial
Occasionally the bereaved person will not accept that their spouse or other loved one has died; instead they will believe that the person is still alive and in hospital. This phase of grieving is sometimes accompanied by 'searching' behaviour. The bereaved person might, for example, visit a spiritualist medium in order to communicate with the dead person. This is not a particularly unusual phenomenon and the problem invariably resolves itself with the bereaved person gradually accepting the loss.

Guilt

The bereaved person may experience feelings of guilt. These may be in relation to things he has said or not said to the deceased. Concern may be expressed about action that should or should not have been taken, particularly in relation to the deceased's welfare. Sometimes the bereaved person will feel guilty about personal criticisms made about the deceased. The mourner may compensate for this guilt by later acknowledging and applauding previously unacceptable aspects of the deceased's behaviour and personality.

Regression

This is not a commonly observed phase of grieving but it does occasionally occur. The mourner resorts to childish, irrational episodes of behaviour which alternate with the reactions of a mature adult. It is important to assist the bereaved person to overcome these problems as failure could result in the problems taking on pathological dimensions.

Depression

One might well expect a bereaved person to be depressed and the readjustment to life following a bereavement is inevitably going to take some considerable time. There are instances, however, when the depression experienced is such that the individual does not seem capable of making the necessary adaptations and continues to be troubled by guilt, other irrational thoughts and may even contemplate the possibility of suicide. When the depression assumes these proportions it is apparent that the individual is in need of professional help and with the consent of the person concerned, appropriate arrangements should be made.

It must be remembered that bereavement, as far as the elderly person is concerned, is likely to be but one of a number of traumatic experiences and that this last personal loss might well result in the individual feeling that life is not worth living. Depression following bereavement can last for a period of up to two years and, during this time, the individual will require very considerable help and support.

Resolution

The bereaved person will ultimately accept the loss and make the adaptations necessary to come to terms with life as it is, rather than what it was or might have been. The individual reorganises commitments and accommodates to a new lifestyle, fully accepting the loss. Rather than continuing to mourn the departure of the loved one, the most valued aspects of the relationship are remembered and comfort is obtained in the knowledge that life has been enriched as a result of the joint affiliation.

Depression in relation to stress

The process of stress involves a series of activities which culminate in an adjustment reaction within the individual.

Fig. 4.3   The process of stress

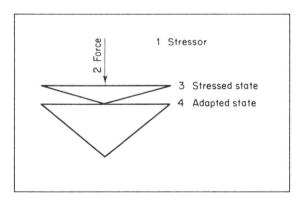

A stressor (1) exerts a force (2) on a body, which becomes stressed (3) and which makes an adaptive response by changing its shape (4).

Stressors

A stressor is an external agent or life event that will produce a stress reaction in an individual. Stressors can be conveniently grouped into four main categories:

1   Physical
2   Psychological

3   Social
4   Economic.

One should, however, recognise that a stressor categorised under one heading is likely to have implications under the others. For example, a physical stressor such as a fall which causes an aged person to break his leg, thus immobilising him, will inevitably result in psychological manifestations, e.g. fear and anxiety. At the same time the injury could result in his becoming socially isolated because of his inability to get out.

At this point, the reader is invited to identify stressors under the headings given and to examine the possible implications insofar as they affect different aspects of the elderly person's life.

The action of stressors inevitably results in physiological as well as psychological stress responses; both are well documented elsewhere. It is important to remember that the physiological response is essentially due to excitation of the sympathetic nervous system and that at times the psychological manifestations will include apprehension, restlessness and irritability, agitation and fear; these are concomitants of anxiety.

The stress process will ultimately culminate in either a socially acceptable form of adaptation or some form of maladaptive response. The fear and anxiety that is often experienced in stress situations often resolves itself without much ado, but occasionally the individual will require some form of help. It is interesting to note that while some stressors evoke a response such as that described above, others, for example death of a spouse, precipitate a depressive reaction. A second point is that some people respond to stress by demonstrating anxiety while others are more likely to become depressed. It is this kind of observation that has tended to lend credence to a medical rather than a psychological approach.

Elements of a stress adaptation model of care

The stress adaptation model of care owes much to the work of Chrisman and Riehl (1974) and Saxton and Hyland (1979). They have undertaken extensive work in its development.

The underpinning rationale assumes that:

1   Man consists of a number of interdependent systems: biological, interpersonal and intrapersonal.
2   Within each system there are a number of subsystems. Some examples are given as follows:

    System: Biological *Subsystems*: Gastrointestinal, cardiovascular, neurological.
    System: Interpersonal *Subsystems*: Sociocultural, interactional, roles.
    System: Intrapersonal *Subsystems*: Selfawareness, self-esteem, personal philosophy.

3   The systems respond to stress situations in either an adaptive or maladaptive manner and accordingly, the individual will demonstrate healthy development or impaired functioning.
4   The different systems also interact with one another and with the environment and this dynamic activity further determines the way in which the individual develops.
5   Development takes place along a continuum from conception to death and is continually being influenced by previous experiences.
6   Adaptation, which may be the result of either inherent characteristics or learning, is also likely to be affected by, for example, the person's level of physical, psychological and social maturity. Saxton and Hyland (1979) also refer to the individual experiencing direct adaptation and on occasions, both direct and indirect adaptation.

Direct adaptation occurs as a result of the individual experiencing some form of external or primary stress. The adaptive response to this initial stress may not always be adequate or appropriate and secondary stress reactions may be observed. Secondary stress reactions give rise to indirect adaptations and these are usually maladaptive in nature.

Saxton and Hyland (1979) have suggested that stress can be experienced at different levels. Initially, it is likely to be seen at local level; if not controlled it will spread to involve an organ. At a tertiary level the stress is seen to invade the entire system. An example involving a physical stressor, such as an infection, would be:

1 at a local level, e.g. cystitis. If not checked here, it may spread to
2 organ level, e.g. nephritis. If not checked at organ level
3 the entire system becomes involved, e.g. uraemia.

In terms of mental health this can be interpreted as follows:

Primary stress: e.g. mildly anxious, worries over problems, feels insecure.
Secondary stress: e.g. experiences physical discomfort and palpitations, unable to eat or sleep.
Tertiary stress: e.g. individual uses avoidance strategies (cannot go out, meet people, etc.)

The above is an example of the stress adaptation process with stress affecting the interpersonal system. It should be noted that at the secondary stress stage, indirect adaptation could occur and become cyclical. Should this happen, the nurse would become involved in planning of a programme of care designed to break the cycle (Fig. 4.4, p 50).

In order to do this the nurse would adopt a problem solving approach, identifying with the patient possible stressors and alternative adaptive responses. It is fundamental to the holistic philosophy underpinning a nursing approach to care that the patient is involved throughout, assisting in elucidating problems, discussing priorities and examining alternative solutions.

The next step is to define the 'key' problems. These are problems of major concern inasmuch as they are likely to trigger off other secondary problems. It follows that if the 'key' problems are identified and resolved, then the secondary problems are unlikely to occur.

Examples of key and secondary problems

The following problems may be expressed by a patient, in non-priority order:

1 feels insecure
2 lacks friends
3 is anxious
4 is not dealing with his personal care
5 suffers from insomnia
6 has lost his appetite
7 feels threatened.

From the above list, two key problems can be identified since they give rise to the other secondary problems:

1 insecurity (interpreted as low self esteem)
2 feels threatened (interpreted as lack of assertiveness).

It should be noted that amongst the commonly recurring key problems, low self esteem, lack of assertiveness and lack of social skills figure prominently. It is thus important to identify problems falling into these categories because it is possible to design care plans that will often help in their alleviation. The stress adaptation model of nursing care presumes that the nurse has a good knowledge of the problems of stress, causes of it and likely physiological and psychological manifestations. It is also essential that the nurse has insights into the patient's perceptions of his problems, his expectations, i.e. what he wants out of life, how he sees his future and what his own plans are. The nurse can then examine with the patient what he wants to achieve, as against that which is realistically possible in the light of all the facts.

It is proposed by Saxton and Hyland that nursing interventions, e.g. offering support by staying with the patient and giving information, can be made at different levels of psychological and physiological adaptation. The ability of the nurse to plan care in accordance with this notion, however, will depend on the nurse's knowledge of how the stress adaptation cycle is likely to develop and the nursing interventions that can be used in either constraining it or in assisting the individual to make a healthy adaptation. The levels of intervention identified are shown in Table 4.3, p 51.

Fig. 4.4 The stress adaptation process

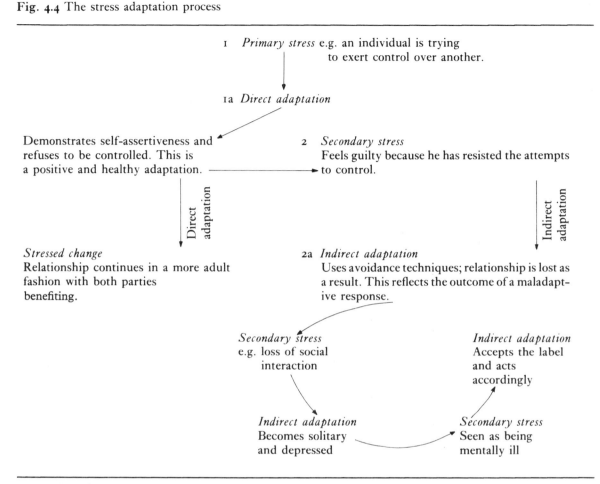

1   *Primary stress* e.g. an individual is trying
    to exert control over another.

1a *Direct adaptation*

Demonstrates self-assertiveness and
refuses to be controlled. This is
a positive and healthy adaptation.

2   *Secondary stress*
    Feels guilty because he has resisted the attempts
    to control.

Direct adaptation

Indirect adaptation

Stressed change
Relationship continues in a more adult
fashion with both parties
benefiting.

2a *Indirect adaptation*
    Uses avoidance techniques; relationship is lost as
    a result. This reflects the outcome of a maladapt-
    ive response.

Secondary stress
e.g. loss of social
interaction

Indirect adaptation
Accepts the label
and acts
accordingly

Indirect adaptation
Becomes solitary
and depressed

Secondary stress
Seen as being
mentally ill

NB   The secondary stress indirect adaptation may be of a cyclical or spiralling nature; in either case nursing
intervention is indicated.

History

Mr. Samuel Parry is seventy-eight years old. He
is a retired schoolteacher and lives alone as his
wife died two months ago. He has a son, Thomas,
who is married and lives in Chester. His daughter, Helen, who is also married, lives ten miles
away. She has three children, the youngest of
whom is six years of age.

Assessment

Saxton and Hyland (1979) do not provide a clear
cut framework for assessment. They point out

Table 4.3 Levels of intervention

Level		Purpose	Example	
			Physical	*Psychological*
1	Support	Nursing action is aimed at assisting the patient in coping with very basic physical and psychological problems	Assisting patient with feeding and carrying out personal hygiene	Staying with the patient and giving information
2	Limit	Nursing interventions designed to contain the problem, thus limiting its spread and effects	Applying pressure to a haemorrhaging wound	Giving information and explaining
3	Alter	Intervention at this level is aimed at reducing the overall effects of the problem	Sitting the patient with respiratory distress up in bed	Use of relaxation techniques
4	Interrupt	Nursing care is aimed at preventing new problems	The patient at risk from pressure sores is turned frequently	Patient is protected from having to make decisions
5	Supplement	Care is aimed at protecting the patient in potentially life threatening situations	The use of artificial respiration	Learning socially acceptable ways of coping with aggression

that:

> The problem of assessing the patient's adaptive level is difficult and requires that the nurse use individual's specific complaints, level of development, past history, as well as laboratory reports and personal observations.

They stress that the assessment process must be ongoing and flexible and should highlight the area of primary concern. They go on to say that:

> each patient will present a different pattern of needs, and care can be individualised only when directed toward the specific pattern that each patient demonstrates.

The importance of getting the assessment phase right cannot be overemphasised. However, it will be appreciated from the above that much depends on the skills, knowledge and attitudes of the nurse. In the following care study, an attempt has been made to use an assessment process that highlights the areas of concern for a particular individual.

Physical health

Mr. Parry's physical health has been generally good for a man of his years. He does have some arthritis in his left hip which makes walking slow and painful at times. He has, however, always tried to keep himself fit. He does not smoke and only drinks on social occasions. His appetite has been good.

Four months ago, Mr. Parry saw his general practitioner about his arthritis and at that time it was discovered that his blood pressure was raised considerably. He was prescribed medication which was effective in its control.

Mental health

Mr. Parry's mental health had previously been good. He was alert and kept up-to-date with current affairs. A keen photographer, he has continued to do his own developing and printing until very recently. He is a member of the local photographic society.

Social situation

Mr. Parry lives in a neat semi-detached house in a pleasant residential area in North London. He cannot do as much about the house now as he used to, and finds it difficult to cope with washing, cooking and other domestic chores.

He was extremely close to his wife. He does not get on very well with his son, however, and only sees him two or three times a year. Mr. Parry's daughter visits twice a week.

Recent events

Mr. Parry's wife died suddenly two months ago. He took his loss very well at the time. Everyone rallied round and assisted with the funeral arrangements. Relatives and friends tended to withdraw after about two weeks. Close neighbours were extremely supportive and friendly towards him.

Ten days ago, these neighbours went away on a winter holiday. His daughter came to visit following an absence of a fortnight due to the illness of her children. She found:

1   Milk on the step, newspapers and post lying untouched on the hall floor.
2   Her father sitting motionless and staring into space in an extremely cold room. He was very cold to the touch.
3   He had not eaten, in fact there was no food in the house.
4   Her father was unkempt and dirty.
5   The house was dirty and beginning to smell.

After a few minutes Mr. Parry spoke for the first time, asking his daughter to make some tea and for her to give a cup to Mother upstairs.

By this time, Helen was feeling very upset and extremely guilty. She knew that she would not be able to accommodate her father in her own home and, at the same time, recognised that daily visiting would be out of the question. She started to bemoan the fact that there seemed little that could be done and questioned the use of having a 'Welfare State'. She ultimately rang her general practitioner demanding some action.

The general practitioner contacted a community psychiatric nurse who came to make an initial assessment of the situation. It was decided that Mr. Parry should be admitted to hospital.

A care plan based on a Stress Adaptation model

Following a nursing assessment of the patient, the major primary and secondary patient problems were identified. The precipitating stressors were also postulated (see Table 4.4, p 53).

When the problems are ranked in order of priority it is evident that hypothermia will take precedence because of its life threatening nature. Nursing interventions will therefore be planned at the fifth, i.e. supplementary, level.

It can also be established from the list that a number of the problems occur as a result of either bereavement or unresolved grief. Bereavement and grief are not the same. Bereavement implies a loss, while grief is an emotional process that under normal circumstances is likely to occur following such a loss.

The two primary problems identified are:

1   denial resulting from unresolved grief
2   loss of self esteem.

A third problem, previously of less significance, has been exacerbated as a result of Mr. Parry having to do more for himself; this is his lack of mobility and pain brought about by arthritis.

Documentation

Documentation of nursing care should be presented in such a way that the significant features of the nursing history, patient assessment, actual and potential patient problems, associated nursing problems, nursing prescriptions and evaluation procedures are readily discernible. It is necessary to identify patient problems and relate them to the presence of stressors. Care plans must state what nurse/patient activities will be necessary in order to normalise or reduce the stress state. The presentation of written information should be lucid and concise and reflect the model of care being used.

Table 4.4 Mr. Parry's assessment

Problem	Stressor(s)	Primary/Secondary
Walking, slow and painful	1 Degeneration of hip joint	Primary to arthritis
	2 Change in role	Secondary to bereavement
Cannot do household chores or cook	1 Loss of mobility	Secondary to arthritis
	2 Change in role	Secondary to bereavement
Loss of companionship of wife	Unresolved grief	Primary to grief
Hypothermia	Lack of heating, food and mobility	Secondary to bereavement
Lack of attention to personal hygiene	Loss of volition and self esteem	Secondary to grief
House is dirty	Lack of volition Loss of mobility	Secondary to grief
Denial of wife's death	Unresolved grief	Primary to grief
Support system failed	Bereavement	Secondary to bereavement

Fig. 4.5 Problems associated with bereavement and grief

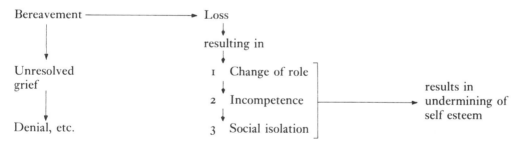

Caring objectives

Caring objectives may be described as being either nurse or patient centred. Ideally they should be mutually negotiated, that is to say both the patient and the nurse will have shared in agreeing the decisions leading to the type, emphasis and direction of prescribed therapeutic activities based on assessment information. However, it is often the nurse who will be asked to take responsibility for explaining the available options and clarifying the pros and cons of alternative solutions. Accordingly, it is probably better to identify caring objectives in terms of nursing activities, acknowledging that these will have been agreed previously with the patient, rather than attempting to state desirable but spurious patient outcomes which may or may not have been negotiated. This does not detract from the fact that it may be necessary to include certain specific patient objectives in the care plan. These should be incorporated as required, e.g. the patient might keep a daily diary in which he indicates his level of mood. Appropriate objectives would be:

1   *As a priority*: to assist the patient in the restoration of his normal body temperature over a period of twenty-four hours.
2   *In the short term*: to protect the patient from the problems of decision-making.
3   *In the mid and long term*: to enable the patient to grieve; to help the patient in restoring his self esteem; to enable the patient to reconstruct his life as he sees it; to assist the patient with exercises designed to increase his range of mobility.

The care plans must indicate how these goals are going to be achieved and which nurse is to be accountable for ensuring that the plans are put into action.

Nursing interventions

Example *1*   Assisting Mr. Parry to grieve

Nurse Smith or her deputy will work through the following progressive regime.
(**NB**   Not all the stages are identified in this example and it will be for the nurse to decide when to progress from one stage to the next.)

1.1   Talk to Mr. Parry about aspects of his life prior to his bereavement.
1.2   Suggest looking at photographs which include pictures of his wife, talk about them and facilitate reminiscences.
1.3   Focus on feelings of anger and guilt and allow Mr. Parry to express his emotions as he determines. This leads to acceptance of his wife's death.
1.4   Encourage him to examine future possibilities and to make decisions of ranging complexity.
1.5   Invite him to write about his feelings and undertake a daily self assessment of his mood.
1.6   Emphasise positive aspects of his feelings and actions rather than negative ones.

Designated nurses will report on progress at each stage of the programme and indicate when Mr. Parry is ready to progress to the next stage.

Example *2*   Helping Mr. Parry to restore his self esteem

On a daily basis, Nurse Smith or her deputy will:

2.1   Negotiate small achievable goals with Mr. Parry, e.g. making snacks and drinks, washing items of clothing.
2.2   Endeavour to ensure success.
2.3   Give praise for trying as well as for achievements.
2.4   Talk about the value of success and what it will enable him to achieve in the future.
2.5   Maintain a record of progress and report back at the weekly case conference.

Evaluation criteria

Evaluation of the care programme will be in terms of:

1   Achievement of the stated objectives
2   Comparison of baseline measurements taken on admission with the degree of improvement demonstrated at pre-determined intervals
3   Feedback from relatives.

Example *1*   Hypothermia

Mr. Parry's body temperature will show a gradual rise over a period of twenty-four hours until his central core temperature reaches 37°C.

Example *2*   Unresolved grief

Mr. Parry will start passing through the stages of grieving, e.g. he will be able to acknowledge his wife's death and deal with her personal effects.

Example *3*   Loss of self esteem

The following should be considered:

a)   Self evaluation by Mr. Parry. The patient indicates his present level of self esteem,

Fig. 4.6 Mr. Parry's self-evaluation

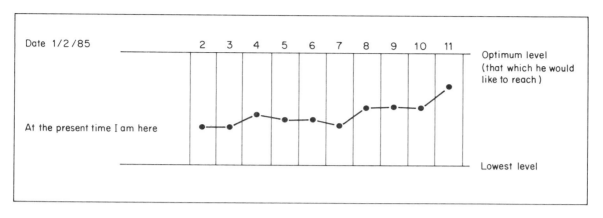

comparing it with his lowest level, and the level he wishes to attain (Fig. 4.6)

b) His ability to involve himself in self care, in particular his physical appearance

c) His ability to make decisions, using a graded scale in order to indicate those ranging from the very simple, e.g. deciding what to eat or drink, to decisions relating to the disposal of his wife's belongings.

Critique of the Stress Adaptation model

The theoretical model on which the Saxton and Hyland approach to care is based suggests that adaptation takes place at three discrete levels: local, organ and system. This kind of compartmentalisation may be acceptable for some physical problems but problems of a more psychological nature cannot be accommodated in this way. The first concern then is that the model is not suited for psychological care, and that its resulting emphasis on the physical could well cause psychological manifestations to be ignored.

The second concern is about the levels of intervention. It is clear that the first intervention is suggested at the 'support' level; however, there

is a need for an earlier stage. Surely there should be a primary preventative level at which the nurse is concerned with health education. It is worthwhile examining the model in light of the Nursing Competencies (a and b) in the Nurses, Midwives and Health Visitors Rules Approval Order 1983: 'advise on the promotion of health and the prevention of illness' and 'recognise situations that may be detrimental to the health and well being of the individual'.

The Chrisman and Riehl (1974) model also provides a basis for the planning of physical care at a secondary or tertiary level; it does however seem to have evolved along unnecessarily complex lines. They introduce the nurse to terms which seem to be of spurious value, e.g. stress quotient, objective/subjective ratio. The reader might like to consider these terms along with a number of others which are used in the original text, deciding on their degree of usefulness.

Chrisman and Riehl refer to their model as the Systems Developmental Stress model. While there is no doubt that a holistic approach to care is intended, the division of man into systems and subsystems could result in nurses thinking in terms of discrete system entities rather than whole individual patients. This is the antithesis of what holism is about and could result in regressive nursing behaviour.

At the present time models of care which were designed primarily with physical care in mind are being stretched to accommodate the needs of those with psychosocial problems. These models tend to concentrate on the activities carried out by nurses and neglect the patient's involvement in their own care which, as far as the psychiatric patient is concerned, is absolutely essential. It is axiomatic in terms of humanistic philosophy that patients should participate in the decision making processes which affect their own care, but in practice the extent of the patient's involvement is rarely reflected in the care plans. Accordingly, while there are benefits to be gained from existing models of care for those whose problems are essentially of a physical nature, there is a need to consider a completely different approach for those with mental illness.

One such approach might start with an examination of why psychiatric patients are seen as being 'ill' in the first place. The common problem shared by mentally ill patients is that of having difficulty in either establishing or maintaining interpersonal relationships. In order for this problem to be surmounted, the individual must be aided in the restructuring of his methods of approach to the formation of interpersonal relationships. It should be noted, however, that the only person who can actually do the restructuring is the patient. While the nurse might be able to help the patient to gain an understanding of some of the related problems, the actual restructuring must of necessity be that of the patient's own choosing and he must undertake it himself.

Finally, it is clear that the model has been made to fit this history to an unwelcome extent, and its widespread use in psychiatric nursing is not envisaged. Having said that however, the model has presented a rational approach to the problems of care and it could be of value in planning the care of those individuals with problems of a predominantly physical nature.

References

Cadoret RJ, Winoku G & Clayton RJ   1970   Family History Studies: VII Manic depressive disease versus depressive disease. *British Journal of Psychiatry*, **116**: 625–635.

Chrisman M & Riehl J   1974   The systems developmental stress model. In: Riehl JP & Roy C (Eds) *Conceptual models for nursing practice*. Appleton-Century-Crofts, Norwalk.

Clare A   1980   *Psychiatry in dissent. Controversial issues in thought and practice*. 2nd Ed. Tavistock, London.

English House Condition Survey.   1976 & 1981   Dept of Environment.

Gerber I *et al.*   1975   Anticipatory grief and aged widows and widowers. *Journal of Gerontology*, **30**: 225–229.

Goble IWJ   1979   An illness that keeps on recurring. *Nursing Mirror*, February: 41–43.

Godber C   1978   Half of the elderly suicides see a GP in their last week of life. *Modern Geriatrics*, August: 24–29.

Great Britain: Statutory Instrument   1983   Nurses, midwives and health visitors rules approval order No. 873. HMSO, London.

Greenblatt   1978   The grieving spouse. *American Journal of Psychiatry*, **135**: 43–47.

Holmes TS & Holmes TH   1970   Short term intrusions into life-style routine. *Journal of Psychosomatic Research*, **14**: 121–132.

Kiev A   1972   *Transcultural psychiatry*. Free Press, New York.

Pollitt J   1978   The depressed patient. *The Practitioner*, **220**: 205–212.

Richter JJ   1984   Crisis of mate loss in the elderly. *Advances in Nursing Science*, July: 45–54.

Rowe D   1985   We are both the helpless prisoner and the cruel jailor. *The Listener*, **7.2**: 8–9.

Sarabin TR   1969   Sociology of conflict. *Contemporary Psychology*, **14**, 3: 186.

Saxton DF & Hyland PA   1979   *Planning and implementing nursing interventions: stress and adaptation applied to patient care*. 2nd Ed. CV Mosby, St. Louis.

Social trends   1985   No. 15. HMSO, London.

Stern K, Williams GM & Prados M   1951   Grief reactions in later life. *American Journal of Psychiatry*, **108**: 289–295.

Szasz TS   1974   *The myth of illness*. Granada, London.

5

The problem of confusion: an examination of Roper's Activities of Living model

Mary Watkins

This chapter demonstrates the use of Roper *et al.*'s model by tracing the nursing care of Mrs. Mary Jones, who presented with a history of increasing confusion, memory loss and urinary incontinence.

The elderly mentally ill assessment ward to which she was admitted was organised into four nursing teams, each headed by a leader who was a qualified nurse responsible for planning and coordinating the nursing care of patients allocated to that team. The other nurses within the team consisted of post-registration nurses, basic student nurses, part-time enrolled nurses and nursing auxiliaries. Altschul (1980) calls this method of planning nursing a 'team approach'. She suggests that patients benefit from this method because they are expected to adjust only to a small number of nurses whilst receiving skilled nursing care. The importance of this point will be demonstrated later.

Selection of nursing model

A nursing model is merely a representation of what nursing is considered to be (Riehl and Roy 1982). It is important to select an appropriate model for the nature of nursing that the person may require. Failure to match nursing model and patient could result in some of the patient's needs not being recognised.

The team leader decided to use an 'activities of living' model of nursing as a framework for managing Mrs. Jones' care. Mrs. Jones presented with a history of confusion, gradual memory loss and urinary incontinence, thus being unable to maintain her normal lifestyle. Yet, as for most elderly patients, on admission the ultimate goal of nursing care was for her to return home.

It is suggested that the Activities of Living model described by Roper *et al.* (1980) provides a suitable framework for the organisation of a patient's nursing needs, while highlighting the need for promoting patient independence. Rule (1976) recognises that it is essential to encompass the physical, emotional and social needs of elderly patients. Roper's model emphasises the physical aspects of care, and so this should be taken into account when planning nursing care to ensure that other needs are also met.

Other models may highlight psychological and social needs more appropriately (Roy 1982). While accepting this fact, it is considered that Roper's model is especially useful in an area where, by tradition, high ratios of untrained staff are employed. The reason for this is that the model uses clear, concise language which is easier to explain and understand than that of most other conceptual frameworks. In addition, it is recognised that physical care of the elderly mentally ill has been overlooked in the past (Robb 1967) and a model which may preclude such negligence in the future addresses these deficits.

Activities of Living model

The model was first described by Roper (1976) and modified by Roper, Logan and Tierney (1980). It suggests that we all undertake certain activities during our everyday lives, albeit in a very individualistic way. In order to fulfil these activities, three types of behaviour are utilised; preventing, comforting and seeking. For example, a person may prevent herself falling out of bed by tucking in the blankets, thus maintaining a safe environment. Similarly, when very tired, people comfort themselves by going to bed early with a hot drink. Seeking activities include those of finding out new information and learning new skills. The model of living is concerned with the whole of a person's life from conception to death. However, because there are periods in life when a person cannot perform the activities of living unaided, for example as a baby or when ill, each person is said to have a dependent/independent continuum for each activity along which movement can take place (Fig. 5.1).

Fig. 5.1. Model of Living after Roper, Logan & Tierney (1980)

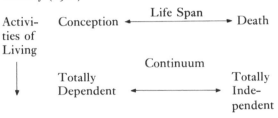

This way of thinking about living is transferred to nursing in order to provide a framework for practice.

Roper (1976) states that the term 'activities of living' was selected in preference to that of 'basic human needs' as the word 'need' has a negative connotation and the word 'activities' has a positive connotation even when a person requires help.

Roper (1976) emphasises the need for nurses to use the concept of continua for activities of living so that each patient is at his maximum level of independence. This enables the nurse to plan for the patient's normal activities to be followed, so that a period of illness is continuous with the rest of the patient's life and not a 'time out' experience. In other words, the nurse should endeavour to encourage the person to follow his normal living pattern even when unwell.

The seeking, comforting and preventing activities described in the model of living are also reflected in the model for nursing. Examples of

these as applied to Mrs. Jones will be described later.

In addition, the dependent component of nursing is described, which is derived from the patient's seeking activities. The patient seeks medical help and as a consequence may require nursing. This dependent part of the role, Roper *et al.* argue, is that which results because of another's prescription, for example giving a patient medication. In Roper's original work, this component was labelled 'administering medical prescription' and was changed presumably in order to encompass activities carried out by the nurse on the request of others.

Neither label appears to be entirely satisfactory in that both terms, dependence and administering medical prescriptions, imply a hand-maiden role for the nurse, rather than one which demands interdependent decision-making. Thus the term 'facilitating' is used in the place of the dependent component of nursing. Both preventing and comforting express an active component of nursing and it is suggested that facilitating does also. Thus a patient seeks medical help, is prescribed medication and the nurse facilitates the patient to take this medication by administering it as prescribed.

Activities of Living using a model of nursing: application of the problem-solving approach

It is stressed here that a problem-solving approach to the practice of nursing fits with this model. The four stages of the nursing process can be utilised to assess, plan, implement and evaluate individual patients' care.

Detailed assessment

Mrs. Mary Jones, aged 69, was admitted from home with a medical diagnosis of acute confusional state. On admission, Mrs. Jones was accompanied by her married daughter, Mrs. Jane Colley.

Mrs. Jones and her daughter lived some 17 miles apart in neighbouring country villages. Mrs. Jones' initial assessment interview (Millar 1981) was conducted by the team leader and involved both Mrs. Jones and her daughter. The initial interview is seen as important by the nurse because it is where communication begins between patient and nurse. The Activities of Living model of nursing was used as the assessment framework to establish the patient's ability to cope. Importance was placed on the initial assessment of Mrs. Jones' needs because an accurate assessment is a vital baseline from which to organise care (McFarlane and Castledine 1982). The non-verbal interviewing skills concerned with relaxing the interviewee by sitting at the same level, maintaining short periods of eye contact, smiling and nodding encouragement were utilised (Argyle 1978).

Similarly, verbal interviewing skills such as clear concise questioning and encouraging Mrs. Jones to ask for information and to express her feelings were employed. The nurse offered Mrs. Jones and her daughter tea during the interview but this was refused and the refusal was respected.

The assessment included obtaining the following information:

1 Personal (biographical) data
2 Data concerning Mrs. Jones' normal routines and level of dependence/independence for each activity of living
3 Identification of strengths and weaknesses
4 Actual and potential problems.

Personal Data

The nurse wished to establish certain personal data, such as Mrs. Jones' next of kin, whether she lived in a flat or house, in order to identify any possible problems (Appendix 1). Similarly, it was considered necessary to establish her religious beliefs in case this should influence her activities of living while in hospital. Whilst it is recognised that information should be collected from the patient whenever possible (McFarlane and Castledine 1982), this is not always practicable. In Mrs. Jones' case it quickly became clear that

whilst she could contribute information, she was unable to give coherent answers to specific questions. The information which she chose to supply herself, such as the fact that her right leg was painful, was received positively by the nurse and recorded. Specific questions, for example how long Mrs. Jones had lived alone, were addressed to Mrs. Colley.

Mrs. Colley had taken the trouble to accompany her mother to hospital and was keen to be involved in her care. The nurse felt it appropriate therefore to include Mrs. Colley in the inverview.

The interview lasted for 40 minutes and during this time, it became apparent that Mrs. Jones had considerable difficulty concentrating. She constantly stood up and asked where she was, stating that she wanted to go home. Her daughter and the nurse explained on several occasions that she was in hospital and this temporarily reassured her. However, within a very short span of time, approximately 5 minutes, she became anxious again and appeared to have forgotten what had been said to her previously.

The assessment strategy suggested by Roper *et al.* was attempted by establishing Mrs. Jones' normal routines concerning the activities of living, and her present level of ability to accomplish each one. It is suggested that, by identifying these differences, nurses can plan the patient care to fit with the individual's routine. An example in Mrs. Jones' situation is given below.

Fig. 5.2 Normal routines and level of dependence/independence.

Personal cleansing and dressing	*Usual routines/what she can/cannot do independently*
	Clean and fastidious, but cannot manage bathing alone
	Present situation No longer washing herself or keeping clothes clean Sleeping in day clothes Difficulty in dressing in sequence

Mrs. Colley tried hard to answer the questions but feared that she may not always be answering accurately. The reason for this, she explained, was that prior to her mother's recent illness she usually visited her once a week, thus she was not certain about how much her mother ate or how long she slept at night. The nurse reassured Mrs. Colley by explaining that Mrs. Jones' behaviour would be closely observed in the ward, providing additional insight into her state of health, and that no firm conclusions would be drawn from Mrs. Colley's information alone. On this occasion, the nurse felt that in order to make an accurate assessment of Mrs. Jones' ability to fulfill her activities of living, close observation of her behaviour should be made during the first 24 hours of her admission.

During this discussion Mrs. Jones' impatience with long conversations became apparent as she fiddled with her clothes and avoided eye contact. As a result of the nurse's awareness of these factors, she had several short conversations with Mrs. Jones rather than one long one, thereby avoiding distressing her further.

This information was conveyed to staff on the other shift who adopted similar strategies. The following morning, the team leader collated all the information gained from both the initial interview and the period of observation using the Activities of Living framework (Appendix 1).

Identification of Strengths and Weaknesses
At this stage, Mrs. Jones' strengths and weaknesses were identified in order to ensure that her nursing care was organised to promote maximum independence. The strengths included the ability to read the headlines of the newspaper when asked to and she demonstrated adequate hearing and vision. Similarly, she was mobile with a walking stick and had no known history of falling. Mrs. Jones' weaknesses were identified in terms of the activities of living she was finding difficult to fulfill unaided. These included memory loss, confusion, difficulty in dressing, painful right leg, breathlessness on exertion and inadequate dietary intake.

Actual and Potential Problems
The deficits in Mrs. Jones' ability to look after herself were then listed in terms of actual and potential problems. Actual problems are those which are clearly identifiable and include inhibited mobility and incontinence of urine. Potential problems are those which the nurse predicts may happen, based on her professional knowledge.

An example of the actual and potential problems Mrs. Jones presented within the activity of personal cleansing and dressing is given below.

The *actual* problems were:
Inability to wash hair and get in and out of the bath.
The *potential* problems include:
Skin breakdown and infection due to poor hygiene.
Reduced self esteem due to reduced ability to maintain personal hygiene and appearance.

To aid nursing assessment, the Norton (1962) pressure area calculator was used which indicated that Mrs. Jones was at risk of developing pressure sores as she scored 12. This scale was designed originally for use with geriatric patients and is a useful aid for the nurse working with elderly people.

A written assessment was produced by the team leader from the data collected (Appendix 1).

Planning

In order to plan Mrs. Jones' care effectively, the team leader considered the aetiology of confusion and appropriate nursing research.

Confusion
The aetiology of confusion is documented in order to demonstrate how the nurse used this both to define Mrs. Jones' potential problems and plan her care.

The term 'confusion' refers to symptoms and signs which indicate the patient is unable to think with his customary clarity and coherence (Lishman 1980). Confused states can be both acute and chronic. Acute confusional states are generally abrupt in manifestation and the majority are reversible when the underlying pathology can be remedied. In contrast, chronic confusional states generally begin insidiously and their

Table 5.1 Causes of acute organic reactions in the elderly (after Lishman 1980)

1 *Degenerative*—presenile or senile dementias complicated by infection, anoxia etc.
2 *Space occupying lesions*—cerebral tumour
3 *Infection*—encephalitis, meningitis, meningovascular syphilis
4 *Vascular*—arteriosclerotic dementia
5 *Metabolic*—uraemia, liver disorder, electrolyte disturbances
6 *Endocrine*—myxoedema, hypoglycaemia
7 *Toxic*—alcohol; i.e. Wernicke's encephalopathy, delirium tremens; drugs, i.e. prescribed medications, such as digoxin, antiparkinsonian agents
8 *Anoxia*—bronchopneumonia, congestive cardiac failure, cardiac dysrhythmias
9 *Vitamin lack*—thiamine (Wernicke's encephalopathy), B_{12} and folic acid deficiency

Table 5.2 Causes of chronic organic reactions in the elderly (after Lishman 1980)

1 *Degenerative*—senile dementia, arteriosclerotic dementia, Alzheimer's disease
2 *Space occupying lesions*—cerebral tumour
3 *Infection*—acute and chronic encephalitis
4 *Vascular*—cerebral arteriosclerosis
5 *Epileptic*—'epileptic dementia'
6 *Metabolic*—uraemia, liver disorder
7 *Endocrine*—hypo/hyperparathyroidism, hypoglycaemia
8 *Toxic*—'alcoholic dementia' and Korsakov's psychosis
9 *Anoxia*—anaemia, congestive cardiac failure, chronic pulmonary disease, post-anaesthetic poisoning, carbon monoxide poisoning, post-cardiac arrest
10 *Vitamin lack*—lack of thiamine, B_{12}, folic acid

history commonly extends over several months (Lishman 1980).

Table 5.1 demonstrates acute confusional states that can be caused by physiological (organic), psychological and sociological factors. For clarity, the organic causes are separated from the psychological and sociological ones. However, all these factors are inextricably united and confusional states often arise when two or more factors combine, i.e. poor social conditions leading to infection and thus to a confusional state.

Table 5.2 demonstrates the common causes of chronic organic reactions in the elderly. Some of the causes listed, e.g. hypoparathyroidism and tumours, can produce both acute and/or chronic confusional states. Clearly, confusional states that are purely physiological in origin require different nursing intervention from those which are psychological or sociological in origin. In the case of a patient with Alzheimer's disease, his physiological state is unlikely to improve and thus the nursing plan to aid him to fulfill his activities of living must take this into account. Similarly, a patient presenting with an acute confusional state due to anoxia resulting from bronchopneumonia requires a nursing plan

which is based on the expectation of reversing the psychopathology. The long term aim for the latter patient would be to resume his previous lifestyle (with appropriate changes to prevent further illness if necessary), the former's long term aim being to maximise independence within his capabilities. It is hoped that this discussion indicates the need for nurses to have a thorough understanding of the aetiology of disease before planning care.

Psychological and social causes of confusion in the elderly can be closely linked. Some common factors are listed in Table 5.3 and their interdependence demonstrated.

Care planning based on nursing research and a hierarchy of needs

Using the knowledge regarding causes of confusion, Mrs. Jones' care (Appendix 2) was organised so that emphasis was placed on the nurse guiding and supporting Mrs. Jones, acting only when absolutely necessary, for example when faecally incontinent, by helping her to clean herself. Wherever possible, the causes of Mrs. Jones' difficulties were identified so that appropriate intervention was planned (McFarlane and

Table 5.3 Some common sociological and psychological factors which contribute to the onset of confusional sates in the elderly (after Lishman 1980)

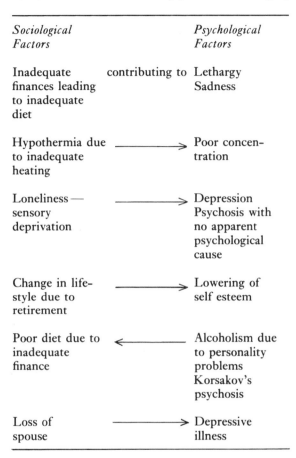

Sociological Factors		Psychological Factors
Inadequate finances leading to inadequate diet	contributing to	Lethargy Sadness
Hypothermia due to inadequate heating	⟶	Poor concentration
Loneliness — sensory deprivation	⟶	Depression Psychosis with no apparent psychological cause
Change in lifestyle due to retirement	⟶	Lowering of self esteem
Poor diet due to inadequate finance	⟵	Alcoholism due to personality problems Korsakov's psychosis
Loss of spouse	⟶	Depressive illness

Fig. 5.3   Maslow's hierarchy of needs (1954)

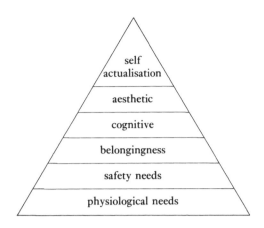

Castledine 1982). It was hoped that a stimulating, rewarding relationship with the nurses would provide an environment in which Mrs. Jones could be independent, the eventual aim being for Mrs. Jones to return to her own home.

Roper *et al.* advocate the use of Maslow's (1954) hierarchy of needs in order to prioritise care. This hierarchy, set out as follows, suggests that until the basic needs are met, at least in part, individuals cannot achieve higher needs.

Mrs. Jones' physiological needs included those of hygiene, hydration and mobilisation. Mrs. Jones was taken to the toilet at frequent intervals to prevent urinary incontinence and a specimen sent to pathology for microculture and sensitivity tests. It was necessary to identify whether Mrs. Jones' incontinence was caused by infection so that treatment could be initiated and the problem thus resolved.

Physical care included giving extra bran (one tablespoon at breakfast) and fluid to reduce incontinence of faeces and constipation. Similarly, mobilisation was encouraged to reduce the risk of deep vein thrombosis. Her right leg was painful due to idiopathic cellulitis. Nursing care involved elevating the leg when Mrs. Jones was sitting and regular application of lanolin cream to prevent skin breakdown. It was thought that an improvement in hydration and diet, coupled with the prophylactic use of oral antibiotics, would reduce the inflammation. Mrs. Jones was also given regular analgesia as prescribed to reduce pain.

While physiological and security needs were emphasised in this early stage of Mrs. Jones' admission, consideration was also given to her need for self esteem. Burton (1976) points out the risk of institutionalisation in mental hospitals and the resultant lack of power for the patient. Thus, Mrs. Jones was given the power to contribute to her own decision making and was verbally rewarded by the nurses for independent behaviour. This process is commonly known as reinforcement. Similarly, the need for Mrs. Jones to become aware of her surroundings and develop a sense of belonging was considered.

These nursing actions focused upon 'reality orientation', a therapy designed to reduce disorientation in confused, elderly people and which attempts to re-orientate them to their environment (Burton 1982). Interventions should be appropriate to the institutional context and to the clients themselves. For example, if Mrs. Jones was found wandering in the early hours, the nurse might say 'Mrs. Jones, it is 5 o'clock in the morning, you are in hospital, I'm a nurse, is there something you need?' Such a statement is client-orientated, enquiring after Mrs. Jones' needs, while appropriate to the institutional context in which the information is given.

Burton (1982) demonstrated that reality orientation may help individuals improve their orientation to the environment, but there is no evidence that it produces any other behavioural changes. It was hoped to orientate Mrs. Jones to the ward and to this end, nursing care was structured using verbal information and spatial orientation (Gilleard *et al.* 1981), the latter intervention involving cardboard signs over doors indicating the toilet, bathroom, nurses' station, sitting room and individual patients' side rooms. Thus, Mrs. Jones' room was clearly labelled. In addition, a date and 'next meal due' board were prominently displayed on the ward. The date board was changed daily before breakfast and the 'next meal due' inserted in the presence of the patients at the end of the previous meal.

As well as reducing disorientation, a second value of reality orientation is that it may provide a bridge on which nurse/patient interaction can be based, therefore increasing such interaction, reported as being infrequent in psychiatry (Altschul 1972).

It was envisaged that, as Mrs. Jones' physical health improved, greater emphasis would be placed on the social and psychological aspects of her care.

Behavioural outcomes and aims of nursing intervention

It is accepted that 'behavioural outcomes' are recommended to identify clearly the aim of nursing actions (McFarlane and Castledine 1982). These outcomes have four components;

1 the person involved (usually the patient)
2 expected behaviour of the person
3 the time in which the behaviour should occur
4 the environmental factors in which this should take place.

An example is:
Eating and drinking
Expected outcome   (1)   Mary Jones
           (2)   will drink 2 litres of fluid
           (3)   every twenty-four hours

These 'expected outcomes' are clearly measurable by the nursing staff. However, these may neglect the affective domain of a patient's care, for example; 'encourage Mrs. Jones to join activities she enjoys'. The enjoyment may only be realised at a particular time on a particular day and not be repeatable. Thus, the expected outcome, 'Mrs. Jones will watch television from 6 pm to 7 pm on Tuesday evenings' may not be useful because on some Tuesdays Mrs. Jones may not feel like doing this. This concept may also help staff to motivate themselves to work with patients who recover slowly or incompletely, whereas using expected outcomes which are not achieved by the patient may result in frustration for all concerned. In addition, it cannot be ignored that the behavioural approach may reduce care to a set of mechanistic steps that miss completely the importance of the developing relationship between patient and nurse.

It soon became clear that Mrs. Jones' care demanded, as a priority, interventions that revolved around comforting, preventing and facilitating.

Preventing interventions included:
Preventing incontinence
Preventing pressure sore development
Preventing inappropriate dressing

Comforting intervention included:
Giving her a diet she likes
Arranging for family photographs to be brought in

Facilitating measures included:
Administering aspirin as prescribed to reduce pain
Taking a mid-stream specimen of urine for culture

Due to Mrs. Jones' acute confusional state she was unable to carry out many activities of living, including elimination, sleeping, personal cleansing and dressing, without support. In this kind of instance, it is necessary for nurses to take over responsibility temporarily in order to ensure patient safety. This tends to result in care plan goals becoming more nurse-centred than patient-centred. The important factor to remember is that nurses should return as much responsibility and independence to the patient as they can, as soon as possible (Roper *et al.*).

Roper *et al.*'s model makes allowances for this kind of nursing care, in that while emphasising the need for patient independence, provision is made for nurses 'acting for' the patient. This sometimes results in nurse-orientated goals such as 'to assess further'. Similarly, interventions can become nurse-centred rather than patient-centred. This is appropriate when a patient is 'dependent' in an activity of living, in that the nurse 'acts' in order to prevent patient deterioration.

To summarise, the main aims of Mrs. Jones' initial care plan were as follows:

1   To plan her care in accordance with Maslow's hierarchy of needs.
2   To promote maximum independence within her capabilities.
3   To assess further her memory span, concentration ability and confusional pattern.
4   To prevent any deterioration in her condition if possible (i.e. skin breakdown, pressure sores).
5   To ensure that the nursing intervention resulted in her hospital stay fitting with her normal routines at home.

To augment planning in this situation, the team leader was influenced by the research that highlights the problems of close relationship with patients (Menzies 1961 and Main 1968). In order to illustrate the importance of this point, these two papers are outlined below.

Research concerning anxiety and conflict in nursing staff
Two papers (Menzies 1961 and Main 1968) are examined, which discuss in detail the anxiety, conflict and stress caused by nursing individual patients. Menzies' work suggests that nursing care is practised in a task-orientated, routine manner in order to protect nurses from the anxiety of close contact with patients. In a similar vein, Main discusses the guilt, depression, anxiety and despair nurses feel when patients only recover very slowly or incompletely. Frequently, nurses cannot reconcile themselves to this failure and they make enormous efforts beyond the call of duty to help these patients. This guilt and resentment is sometimes projected by nurses onto other carers (e.g. doctors, colleagues, relatives), which may affect the quality of care patients actually receive.

It is suggested that an awareness of this research could be of particular value to nurses involved in the care of the elderly mentally disturbed. This group of patients is very often slow to respond to treatment and, as has been demonstrated, may not recover completely. If nurses are aware of their own feelings, these can often be discussed and worked through. Similarly, if a detailed nursing care plan exists, which is shared by all staff, nurses may be able to conduct individualised care without the burden of carrying *individual responsibility* for a patient's care.

How this affected Mrs. Jones' care
The team leader tried to plan realistic goals for Mrs. Jones' care rather than 'ideal' ones which might never be met. Naturally she wished for Mrs. Jones to achieve continence and her nursing aim could have been 'to be continent in one week'. A realistic aim and associated intervention, however, may be to 'prevent Mrs. Jones

from being incontinent by prompting and guiding her to the toilet at certain times'.

By planning care in this manner and recognising that this meets the nurse's needs (i.e. a measure that some intervention is having a satisfactory outcome), the patient's and the nurse's anxiety may be decreased. Nurse anxiety is readily transferred to patients (Menzies 1961), so by reducing this, care may hopefully be improved.

Mrs. Jones' initial care plan is documented in Appendix 2.

Implementation of nursing care

Mrs. Jones' care plan was used as a prescription for nursing care by the whole team, all encouraging her to be as independent as her condition allowed while ensuring that her safety was maintained.

At times Mrs. Jones seemed to enjoy chatting, especially about the war years. However, it quickly became apprent that she could not remember the names of nurses or patients on the ward. Her concentration remained short-lived (approximately 5 minutes) whether she was reading, watching television or conversing.

A mid-stream specimen of urine was obtained on the second day of Mrs. Jones' admission and sent for microculture and sensitivity tests. In addition to the care planned, nurses accompanied Mrs. Jones to the general hospital for a brain scan, where she grew restless waiting, but responded to looking at magazines for short periods.

At night Mrs. Jones responded to the chloral hydrate and slept well. This reduced her distress and the night nurses did not find it necessary to use cot sides at any time.

On the fourth day of admission the pathology department reported that Mrs. Jones had a urinary tract infection. This was sensitive to the antibiotic she had been prescribed by medical staff immediately after the specimen had been collected.

Mrs. Jones' nursing care was evaluated daily but no change in plan was necessary as her condition steadily improved. The nurses did not want to change her plan unless it was vital because Mrs. Jones was anxious and confused and frequent changes in lifestyle are likely to increase this (Lishman 1980, Kreigh & Perko 1979). Also, one of the aims of nursing was to gain an accurate assessment of her memory, confusion and concentration abilities. Constant changes in care could have prevented this by increasing her disorientation.

The daily evaluations were conducted as McFarlane and Castledine suggest; by systematically reviewing the stated patient problems and nursing orders of the care plan at daily report sessions. Lelean (1973) found that report sessions can become a one-way process from sister to nurse. Every effort was made to ensure that all nurses including assistants could voice their opinions in these sessions.

Seven days after admission a comprehensive multidisciplinary team evaluation of Mrs. Jones' health was conducted and the details were as follows.

Multidisciplinary evaluation
Mrs. Jones' urinary tract infection had responded to treatment and her urinary incontinence improved considerably. The nursing staff had observed Mrs. Jones' memory span, confusional state and concentration ability while she had been on the ward. The team summarised this in a handover meeting (Table 5.4) and presented

Table 5.4 Nursing assessment of Mrs. Jones' memory, confusion and concentration ability

Memory span: Can remember her past life well. Unable to learn new names (including her grandchildren). Forgets immediately whether she has eaten or been to the toilet.
Confusional state: Has not accepted that she is in hospital and is not sure where she is most of the time. Is not aware of the time of day, the weather and is unable to answer specific questions. Her mood varies from cheerful to sad for no apparent reason.
Concentration ability: Has not been able to concentrate on any activity including eating, reading, washing, dressing for more than 5 minutes.

it at the multidisciplinary evaluation meeting. Unfortunately, medical examination coupled with the nursing assessment resulted in a diagnosis of irreversible Alzheimer's disease.

Alzheimer's disease is classified as a pre-senile dementia, but cases of late onset are recognised (Lishman 1980). The onset is usually insidious and intellectual deterioration slow and fortunately, the sufferer usually does not realise what is happening (Lishman 1980). Mrs. Jones' presentation fits this classic description in that her daughter admitted that her mother had been unwell for several years 'but it's been very slow and she always seems cheerful'.

There are three main phases of the disease, the first involving failing memory, muddled inefficiency and spatial disorientation. In addition some patients suffer mood disorder in the form of perplexity and agitation. The second phase involves the individual's intellectual and personality deterioration and disturbance in posture and gait (Lishman 1980). Mrs. Jones presented with all these symptoms and was incontinent, which is associated with the third and final phase.

Following the multidisciplinary review of Mrs. Jones' health, a comprehensive formal evaluation of her nursing care was conducted.

Evaluation of care already given and reassessment of nursing needs

An evaluation of Mrs. Jones' nursing care was made by the team leader in conjunction with the rest of the nursing team (Appendix 3). The nursing team felt that the use of Roper *et al.*'s model of nursing provided a useful framework within which to plan Mrs. Jones' nursing. The framework encompassed 'preventing' Mrs. Jones from deteriorating further (e.g. by falling), allowed for 'comforting' in the form of planning a diet similar to that she had at home, and 'facilitating' some degree of recovery from a urinary tract infection and inflamed leg by administering prescribed medication. However, in accepting the diagnosis of Alzheimer's disease, the main aim of Mrs. Jones' nursing care should now focus on encouraging her to be as independent as her capabilities allowed (Pitt 1974).

This aim corresponds to that of the 'activities of living' model. The nursing team decided to reassess Mrs. Jones' needs in order to ensure that her strengths were incorporated into the care plan. It was recognised that, in the initial stages of Mrs. Jones' care, many of the care plan goals had been nurse-centred. It was necessary to reconsider these in order to give Mrs. Jones as much responsibility as possible. However, behavioural outcomes, which included specific time limits, were for the most part considered inappropriate, because of the nature of Mrs. Jones's disease process.

The list of activities of living considered were those described by Roper *et al.* plus those of 'memorising' and 'perceiving'. The reasons for adding these included the fact that Mrs. Jones had difficulty with them and required help. Grant and White (1983) report having to use these categories together with the activities of living when caring for an elderly confused patient. They chose to document these 'psychological factors' separately but the team leader believed they were 'activities of living' in the sense that most people memorise and perceive as a part of life. It may be suggested that these activities could be included within the activity of 'communicating'. However, it is thought that the importance of these activities is reduced by including them under a broad heading. Smith (1980), in a comprehensive psychiatric nursing history and data sheet, gives prominence to the assessment of 'memory' and 'perception' in order to provide a detailed psychological nursing assessment. Accepting Rule's (1976) belief that psychological and social needs are as important as physiological ones, it is considered appropriate to add these categories as separate entities, thereby emphasising their value to the nursing team.

Implementation
A second daily care plan incorporating the above evaluation was drawn up together with Mrs. Jones, the purpose of this being to discuss her own care with her and to provide clear guidelines on how she might spend her day in hospital. It was hoped that, having given her such a plan, she might read it when she was not sure what to do.

The plan was made on a large piece of paper (newspaper size) and stuck to the side of her wardrobe by her bed. She chose blue and red crayons to create it and appeared to enjoy doing so.

Mrs. Jones' care was continued over a ten day period and reviewed daily in the manner described. No change in her care was necessary.

The long term plan for Mrs. Jones' future was discussed with her daughter, the social worker and the medical team. The nurses were aware of Mrs. Colley's distress over her mother's diagnosis and made her especially welcome when she visited the ward. Over a cup of tea, they discussed Mrs. Colley's anxiety at the thought of her mother deteriorating and tried to reassure her by explaining that Mrs. Jones was not distressed herself.

Throughout Mrs. Jones' stay in hospital, the leader encouraged her team to view Mrs. Jones in the context of her family unit. This is particularly important for patients with dementing illnesses who have difficulty making new social contacts due to their failing memory and poor concentration.

Evaluation

Whilst many authorities believe that nursing care plans should be evaluated daily (McFarlane and Castledine 1982), this was not conducted in a formal manner. Mrs. Jones' care was discussed on a daily basis but not altered unless her condition warranted a change in care. Once a week detailed reviews were conducted, the first of which resulted in changes of care. The second review demonstrated that no change was necessary.

During Mrs. Jones' stay on the ward, the following had been achieved:

ACTIVITIES OF LIVING	IMPROVEMENT IN ABILITY
Maintaining a safe environment	Walks safely unaided as shoe velcro mended
Communicating	No obvious improvement
Breathing	Medication controlling this Input/output well controlled
Eating and drinking	Weight reduction 1.6 kg over 7 days Enjoying diet, including sweeteners in tea
Eliminating	1) Constipation and faecal incontinence improved—daily bowel action 2) Urinary incontinence in the day ceased with regular prompting to go to the toilet 3) Urinary tract infection cleared
Personal cleansing and dressing	1) Sacral and skin soreness avoided—no pressure sores 2) Washes and dresses appropriately with assistance
Controlling body temperature	Pyrexia reduced, temperature within normal limits Urinary tract infection, inflammation and pain in right leg eliminated
Mobilising	Can walk freely without pain No deep vein thrombosis occurred
Working and playing	No evident improvement
Expressing sexuality Dying	Not applicable in these terms
Sleeping	Sleeping well after chloral hydrate Agitation reduced, it has not been necessary to use cot sides
Memorising Perceiving	Two activities which are unlikely to improve significantly due to physiological damage

Mrs. Jones was also asked to assess her own improvement, but she found this difficult and was negative about it. Roper (1976) emphasised the importance of patient self assessment in contributing to their own care. The nurses needed to use listening skills because occasionally Mrs. Jones would spontaneously say how she felt she was managing. For example, one day she remarked on the reduction in her incontinence. The nurses' feelings were included in Mrs. Jones' evaluation as it was recognised that patients respond to these. For example, un-motivated nurses result in unmotivated patients (Barton 1976). Some of the nurses expressed frustration at Mrs. Jones' inability to be involved in her care when the whole point of the Roper *et al.* model is for patients to participate in decision making. The team leader pointed out that at least the use of the model gave Mrs. Jones a chance to be involved, even if she did not choose to do so. Further discussion uncovered the feelings of helplessness within the team due to the fact that, despite working so hard with Mrs. Jones, she was unlikely improve signifi-cantly. The Enrolled Nurse said 'I know intel-lectually from the work of Main why I feel this, but it doesn't stop me feeling like it'. The whole team thought that task allocation masked such deep feelings, as reported by Menzies (1961). However, they all agreed that Mrs. Jones had received better care using team nursing and an activities of living model than she would have done using task allocation. When asked to cate-gorise why they felt this, the following statements emerged:

'Well, we tried to give her things she and her daughter said she liked to eat'.

'The plan fitted with her diagnosis in that we changed it when we knew she had Alzheimer's disease. We don't normally do that—just go on writing the Kardex'.

'It made me think "Why does she have this problem?" For example, forgetting, and that made me more patient because I understood the physiology'.

Clearly Mrs. Jones received a comprehensive nursing assessment and care based on promoting her independence. However, some disadvantages of using the Roper model for a patient with confusion were also identified. Without adding the two activities of living 'memorising' and 'perceiving', these vital categories may not have been assessed accurately and appropriate nursing care overlooked. In some respects, therefore, the model had to be adapted to enhance nursing practice. The need to assess additional categories has been documented (Grant and White 1983).

It is hoped that the care plan described demonstrates the importance of altering a nurs-ing model to fit the patient's needs rather than adhering rigidly to a framework at the expense of meeting those needs.

The activities of living model (Roper *et al.* 1980) proved useful in organising the care of a patient suffering irreversible physiological cer-ebral damage in that the nursing staff were able to 'promote maximum independence' within Mrs. Jones' capabilities, appropriately fitting with her defined needs (Pitt 1974).

References

Altschul A 1972 *Nurse patient interaction.* Churchill Livingstone, Edinburgh.

Altschul A 1980 The team approach to psychiatric care. *Nursing Times,* **76**, 18: 797–798.

Argyle M 1978 *The psychology of interpersonal be-haviour.* 3rd Ed. Penguin, London.

Barton R 1976 *Institutional neurosis.* 2nd Ed. John Wright, Bristol.

Barker PJ 1982 *Behaviour therapy nursing.* Croom Helm, London.

Burton M 1982 Reality orientation for the elderly; a critique. *Journal of Advanced Nursing,* **7**, 5: 427–433.

Gilleard C, Mitchell RG & Riordan J 1981 Ward orientation training with psychogeriatric patients. *Journal of Advanced Nursing,* **6**, 2: 95–97.

Grant N & White B 1983 A study in a psychiatric ward using the model for nursing. In: Roper N, Logan W & Tierney A (Eds) *Using a model for nursing.* Churchill Livingstone, Edinburgh.

Kreigh HA & Perko JE 1979 *Psychiatric and mental health nursing.* Virginia-Reston Pub Co.

Langland RM & Pannicucci C 1982 Effects of touch

on communication with elderly confused clients. *Journal of Gerontological Nursing*, 8, 3: 152–155.

Lelean SR 1973 *Ready for report nurse?* Royal College of Nursing, London.

Lishman WA 1980 *Organic psychiatry.* Blackwell, Oxford.

Maslow AH 1954 *Motivation and personality.* 2nd Ed. Harper & Row, New York.

Main T 1968 The Ailment. In: Barnes E (Ed) *Psychosocial nursing.* Tavistock, London.

McFarlane J & Castledine G 1982 *A guide to the practice of nursing using the nursing process.* Mosby, London.

Menzies I 1961 The functioning of social systems as a defense against anxiety. *Tavistock Pamphlet No. 5.*

Millar E 1981 Learning to communicate. *Nursing*, 27: 1197–1199.

Norton D, Exton Smith AN & McLaren R 1962 *An investigation of geriatric nursing problems in hospital.* Churchill Livingstone, Edinburgh.

Pitt B 1974 *Psychogeriatrics: An introduction to the psychiatry of old age.* Churchill Livingstone, Edinburgh.

Robb B 1967 *Sans everything.* Thomas Nelson, London.

Roper N 1976 A model for nursing and nursology. *Journal of Advanced Nursing*, 1, 3: 219–227.

Roper N, Logan W & Tierney A 1980 *The elements of nursing.* Churchill Livingstone, Edinburgh.

Roy C 1982 The Roy Adaptation Model. In: Riehl JP & Roy C (Eds) *Conceptual models for nursing practice.* 2nd Ed. Appleton-Century-Crofts, Norwalk.

Rule JB 1976 Raising standards of care—what can we afford? *Royal Soc of Health Journal*, 96, 5: 204–208.

Smith L 1980 A nursing history and data sheet. *Nursing Times*, 76, 17: 749–753.

Appendix 1
Nursing Information Sheet

HOSPITAL NO:	WARDS	DATE OF ADMISSION: 3/10/84

SURNAME   JONES
FORENAME   MARY ELIZABETH
ADDRESS   17 High Street
　　　　　　Bethlehem
　　　　　　Herts
LIKES TO BE KNOWN AS: Mrs. Jones
DATE OF BIRTH: 6/3/1915
AGE: 69　　**SEX:**   F
MARITAL STATUS: Widow
RELIGION: C of E
NATIONALITY: British

IS PATIENT FORMAL OR INFORMAL?
　　　　　　　　Informal
SECTION

NEXT OF KIN: Mrs. J. Colley (daughter)
ADDRESS: 10 New Road
　　　　　　Addinfon
　　　　　　Herts
TEL. NO.   Addinfon 67895
**PERSON TO CONTACT IN CASE OF
EMERGENCY:**
(if different from above)
ADDRESS:

TEL. NO.

SIGNIFICANT PERSONS IN LIFE
Daughter and two grandchildren; Angus 17 and
Jenny 11

PATIENT'S PROFILE
Height   5 foot 2 in.
Weight   73.6 kgs.
Build   Medium
Complexion   Fair
Hair – Colour   Grey
Eyes – Colour   Green
Marks and Scars   None

T.P.R.—   T. 38.2, P. 78, R. 18
B.P.—   130/85
Urine—   Ketones and protein present

**RELEVANT PSYCHIATRIC AND GENERAL
MEDICAL HISTORY**
Mrs. Jones suffered a depressive illness after the death of
her husband and was successfully treated as an
outpatient in 1980. (Psychotherapy)
Gradual memory loss over last two years.
Asthma as a child.

OCCUPATION AND PAST WORK HISTORY
Retired for nine years—prior to this was Assistant
Manageress in local supermarket
SOURCE OF FINANCE:
Old age pension and work pension

HOME CONDITIONS
Two bedroomed house which she owns.
No central heating but efficient gas fires downstairs.
Upstairs bathroom.
No toilet downstairs.

**COMMUNITY RESOURCES (CPNS
VOLUNTARY AGENCIES)**
Meals on wheels

SPECIAL NURSING OBSERVATION

REASON FOR ADMISSION:
Increased confusion, rapid deterioration over last two
weeks. Urinary incontinence during the day.

PATIENT ASSESSMENT FORM: ASSESSMENT OF ALs

Date

Activity of living AL	Usual routines what he/she can and cannot do independently	Patient's problems actual/potential
Maintaining a safe environment	Usually manages to adhere to safety rules at home, i.e. locks door at night, turns off electricity Unable at present, forgets to turn kettle off Right surgical shoe velcro broken	1) Could fall due to broken shoe 2) Forgets to turn electrical appliances off due to either memory disturbances or confusion
Communicating	Hearing and sight good Watches television and reads a lot when 'fit' Tends to dwell in the past her daughter says, and not interested in the future 'She would rather talk about the war than computers' (Mrs. Colley's words) Normally writes letters and pays bills etc. Present state—has difficulty in concentrating on a conversation. Memory span approximately five minutes. She would like to go home but does not know where she is at present	1) Concentration span short 2) Memory span approximately five minutes 3) Wants to go home 4) Is not aware she is in hospital 5) May become confused about her role if she forgets home and family
Breathing	Breathless on exertion at home, especially when climbing the stairs due to congestive cardiac failure Also becomes breathless when anxious. (Takes digoxin daily—dose not known) and 'water tablets' when necessary (daughter's information)	1) Breathless on exertion or anxiety 2) Obesity Weight 73.6 kgs 3) Potential problem—fluid retention may increase breathlessness
Eating and drinking	Drinks a lot of hot sweet tea at home—3 tsps. of sugar per cup Eats when she feels like it Not fond of fruit or greens but loves starches and sweet things. Her daughter says that she eats less than she used to Well hydrated on admission	1) Diet may be contributing to obesity and causing breathlessness 2) Potential problem of constipation due to inadequate roughage in diet
Eliminating	Was continent of urine and faeces until two weeks ago Daughter then noticed 'wet sheets' and recently 'faecal incontinence' at night—smearing of faeces on the sheets Now incontinent of urine day and night	1) Urinary incontinence 2) Faecal incontinence, smearing 3) Constipation

PATIENT ASSESSMENT FORM: ASSESSMENT OF ALs (continued)

Date

Activity of living AL	Usual routines what he/she can and cannot do independently	Patient's problems actual/potential
Personal cleansing and dressing	Until three months ago clean and fastidious Community nurse visits once a fortnight to help Mrs. Jones bath and wash her hair Her daughter thinks she has stopped washing herself and her clothes between these visits Last night she tried to sleep in her day clothes and did not wash without prompting Cannot dress in sequence—put her bra on top of her dress False teeth need cleaning	1) Cannot manage to bath or wash her hair unaided 2) Forgets or is not motivated to wash self or clothes 3) Cannot dress in sequence without assistance 4) Risk of pressure sores, Norton Scale 12. Skin breakdown 5) Reduced self esteem due to inability to maintain personal hygiene and appearance
Controlling body temperature	Recently Mrs. Jones has been shopping without dressing warmly Mrs. Jones says she often feels cold Temperature 37.2°c on admission—Mrs. Jones right leg is painful, swollen, red and hot	1) Low grade pyrexia 2) Right leg hot and sore to touch 3) Feels the cold 4) Does not always dress appropriately for the weather
Mobilising	Walks well with a walking stick. Has never fallen to daughter's knowledge Mrs. Jones says she would rather sit in a chair than walk as it hurts her left leg	1) Risk of deep vein thrombosis and pressure sores due to sitting still 2) Pain in calf of right leg on exertion due to inflammation/ cellulitis 3) Reduced mobility due to pain
Working and playing	Has retired, normally enjoys watching television and gardening Used to play 'whist' but has stopped going because she says 'I can't concentrate'	1) Risk of social isolation due to difficulty in concentrating
Expressing sexuality	Mrs. Jones' husband died eight years ago. She was depressed at first but Mrs. Colley feels her mother has got over it She usually makes up and wears perfume but has stopped doing this	1) Stopped wearing makeup and scent
Sleeping	Mrs. Jones says she has never worried about sleeping Her daughter thinks she normally sleeps well but wakes early Last night she became agitated, did not sleep well and cried. The night nurses report finding it difficult to comfort her but sweet tea helped to stop her crying	1) Agitated and distressed at night 2) May fall at night if not supervised

PATIENT ASSESSMENT FORM: ASSESSMENT OF ALs (continued)

Date

Activity of living AL	Usual routines what he/she can and cannot do independently	Patient's problems actual/potential
Dying	Mrs. Colley says that she and her mother have discussed death together. Her mother is a practising Anglican and believes in the after life She thinks Mrs. Jones would like to see the chaplain when he visits	

Appendix 2
Nursing Plan Related to ALs

Goals	Nursing Interventions related to ALs	Evaluation
Maintaining a safe environment	Organise for right surgical shoe to be repaired.	Surgical shoe repaired
Mrs. Jones will not fall in hospital	In the meantime use a strong elastic band to secure it. Ensure Mrs. Jones does not walk about when floor is being cleaned. Mop up any spillage promptly to prevent falling.	
Mrs. Jones will not leave electrical appliances on or harm herself with them	Supervise Mrs. Jones if she wishes to make a cup of tea or use any electrical appliance i.e. hairdryer.	Mrs. Jones does not mind being helped with these appliances
Communicating That Mrs. Jones becomes orientated to the ward	1) Ask Mary her name, where she is daily. Inform her of correct answers. Praise her if correct	No improvement in orientation
That Mrs. Jones maintains her identity	Reinforce her role at home. Ask her daughter for family photos to make a family tree to put by her bed. Reinforce her role in the family by making this with her and reminding frequently.	Her daughter has made a 'family tree'. Continue to talk to Mary about family
To further assess concentration and memory span.	Spend regular periods with Mrs. Jones (at least two per shift of ten minutes duration) and establish how long she can concentrate on a conversation and how much recall of it she has.	Initial assessment complete Discontinue

Goals	Nursing Interventions related to ALs	Evaluation
Breathing Patient's respiratory rate will not exceed 25/minute Patient will take at least 2 litres fluid/24 hours	1) Prevent Mrs. Jones becoming exerted, care when getting in and out of the bath. 2) Fluid input/output chart to ensure no excess retention for 48 hours. Intake minimum of two litres/24 hours. Weigh daily.	No evidence of breathlessness or water retention Review weekly
Eating & drinking Patient will not be faecally incontinent Patient will establish regular bowel habits	One tablespoon of bran on cereal. Encourage to sit on toilet and tell her to open bowels. Praise accordingly.	Mrs. Jones has had bowels open daily for three days
Patient's weight will not increase	Substitute sweeteners for sugar in tea. Allow Mrs. Jones sweet puddings and chocolate. Encourage her to eat some fruit and vegetables.	Mrs. Jones says 'I'm happy with what I'm eating'
Eliminating That Mrs. Jones urinary incontinence is reduced	1) Collect and send to lab. middle stream urine specimen for culture and sensitivity. 2) Habit training take to the toilet when requested and at three hourly intervals.	(3/6/85) 1) This has been done 2) Habit training successful in that incontinence reduced except at night
Personal cleansing That Mrs. Jones is clean and tidy and her skin remains intact	1) Assist with washing, encourage independence as much as possible. 2) Allow her to choose clothes and dress herself but verbally show her the order to dress in and see she has warm enough clothes on. 3) Ask if she would like a bath, particularly after incontinence. Do not force if refuses, just assist with washing.	Mrs. Jones will continue to need this help
Controlling body temperature That Mrs. Jones body temperature is reduced within normal range. That her right leg swelling is reduced	1) Mrs. Jones should drink 2 litres/twenty-four hrs to dilute toxins and reduce temperature. 2) Measure temperature four hourly and give prescribed aspirin to reduce both temperature and pain. 3) Elevate right leg on a stool with a cushion when Mrs. Jones is sitting down.	Mrs. Jones drinks without prompting Pyrexia reduced Pain in right leg reduced but still some swelling Discontinue (1) and (2)

Goals	Nursing Interventions related to ALs	Evaluation
Mobilising That Mrs. J. does not develop pressure sores	Encourage Mrs. Jones to walk in the ward every two hours. Ensure that she is washed quickly when incontinent. Move her position in the bed two hourly at night.	No evidence of skin breakdown Walks freely on the ward with her stick
Working & playing That Mrs. Jones is not socially isolated and enjoys her leisure	Encourage Mrs. Jones to join activities she enjoys. This may include watching television, reading and playing card games. Touch Mary gently on the arm when conversing with her.	This has been partially successful
That Mrs. Jones takes initiative	Reward independent behaviour—i.e. when Mrs. Jones walks with her stick without being asked to.	Mrs. Jones has shown some independent behaviour i.e. has walked up and down to the toilet without assistance or prompting
Expressing sexuality Reinforce her family and feminine role	See those in "Communicating". Encourage Mrs. Jones to use make up and scent as appropriate.	Mrs. Jones is not interested in wearing make up or scent at the moment
Sleeping That Mrs. Jones's agitation & distress are reduced at night	Ensure that she is comfortable in bed and ask if she would like a hot drink if she wakes up. Chloral hydrate has been prescribed and should be given at 10 p.m. Please observe closely to see if this reduces agitation. Try not to use cotsides, but if a nurse is unable to sit in the ward this will be necessary. (This is not the chosen method of care as it may increase confusion and regression).	Successful Continue
To assess Mrs. Jones physical & mental state further	Further assessment before discussing "death" or dying with Mrs. Jones and her daughter, unless Mrs. Jones brings the subject up.	Diagnosis of irreversible Alzheimer's disease.

Appendix 3

ACTIVITY OF LIVING	PRESENT SITUATION	LEVEL OF DEPENDENCE	GOAL	PLAN OF CARE
Maintaining a safe environment	Still cannot remember to switch off electrical appliances without prompting Sometimes gets up when floor being cleaned	Basically independent except with electrical goods and wet floors	That Mrs. Jones does not come to any harm	Ensure Mrs. Jones does not walk about when floor being cleaned 10–11 a.m. Supervise Mrs. Jones if she wishes to make a cup of tea or use any electrical appliances
Communicating	Speaks clearly, but loses thread of conversation very easily. Attention span for conversation is short Enjoys reading newspaper Responds to quiet, calm tone when speaking to her. She can evidently hear satisfactorily, and can read without glasses	Attention span short. Can understand requests and general communication	That she converses with her daughter and the nurses. Orientation to her role	When talking with Mary, try to establish how long she can cope with this, i.e. 10 mins. or $\frac{1}{2}$ h and use her family tree to remind her of her role in the family
Breathing	No evidence of breathlessness since admission. Similarly, has not required diuretics	Managing well at present	Respiration to be within 14 & 20/minute	Observe for breathlessness if Mrs. Jones becomes agitated or distressed. Weigh daily to monitor for fluid retention
Eating and drinking	Eats and drinks when asked to Enjoys sweet foods Weight now 72.0 kgs. has lost 1.6 kgs. since admission	Still over weight at 72 kgs.	Weight loss of 1 kg/week for 6 weeks	Continue to substitute sweetener for sugar in tea Allow Mrs. Jones to eat sweet puddings and chocolate Encourage her to eat some fresh fruit and vegetables

ACTIVITY OF LIVING	PRESENT SITUATION	LEVEL OF DEPENDENCE	GOAL	PLAN OF CARE
Eliminating	Has had her bowels open daily for three days. Still some nocturnal urinary incontinence but this has not occurred in the day	Urinary/faecal incontinence reduced in the day, but she forgets to go to the toilet unless asked Nocturnal incontinence	Absence of constipation. Increased level of continence	1) Prompt Mrs. Jones to go to the toilet after meals and take her if she asks to go 2) Praise accordingly 3) Wake her to use commode at 12 and 4 a.m. 4) Continue to put bran on cereal. Mrs. Jones should drink 2 litres of fluid a day
Personal cleansing and dressing	Mrs. Jones forgets to wash, but will do so when asked. She does not like bathing She has difficulty in dressing without being told the order in which to put her clothes on	Unable to manage washing and dressing without verbal prompting Norton Score 12	Independence in washing and dressing Skin remains intact, soft and supple especially on pressure points	1) Wash immediately if incontinent 2) Prompt Mrs. Jones to wash and see she takes all the necessary tools with her (i.e. soap) to the bathroom 3) Supervise her dressing by giving her underclothes first. Allow her to choose what she wears—i.e. skirt/cardigan
Controlling body temperature	Pyrexia reduced. Right leg swelling and redness has subsided Still does not put on coat to go out	Able to maintain temperature in the ward Needs reminding to wear coat outside	Mrs. Jones body temperature to remain above 36°C and below 37°C Right leg improvement to be maintained	1) Remind Mrs. Jones to put warm cardigan on when she leaves the ward 2) Check her right leg daily for signs of redness
Mobilising	Is able to walk freely on the ward with her stick All pain in right leg gone she says No longer wants to sit all day	Independent— can walk freely	Mrs. Jones to maintain her maximum level of independence	Encourage Mrs. Jones to walk unaided except when floor being cleaned

ACTIVITY OF LIVING	PRESENT SITUATION	LEVEL OF DEPENDENCE	GOAL	PLAN OF CARE
Working and playing	Generally enjoys T.V. Cannot concentrate to play board or card games	May become isolated due to difficulty in concentrating	That Mrs. Jones achieves a balance between social interaction and solitude	Encourage to watch and discuss T.V. with nursing staff and other patients
Expressing sexuality	Likes to have her hair washed and set by ward hairdresser	Unable to wash hair unaided	That she expresses satisfaction with her appearance	Book appointment with hairdresser weekly
Sleeping	Sleeps soundly with Chloral Hydrate as prescribed, nocturnal enuresis	Requires medication to sleep. Nocturnal enuresis	That Mrs. Jones sleeps for eight hours a night	Administer medication as prescribed See Eliminating
Dying	See previous care plan re discussion with daughter			If Mrs. Jones wishes to discuss this do so in an honest and open manner
Memorising	Reverts to the past frequently Short term memory very poor which causes her distress	Long term memory good Short term memory poor	Mrs. Jones' stress regarding her memory loss is reduced	Encourage Mrs. Jones to 'chat' about things she remembers, i.e. the war When she forgets something, for example whether she has had lunch, remind her quietly and calmly—touch her arm as you do so
Perceiving	Mrs. Jones is still confused and disorientated in time and place Does not appreciate that she is 'a patient in hospital'	Confusion and disorientation for the majority of the time Thinks she is at home at times	Reduced disorientation	Show her her room, the board which says date etc. Do not reinforce confusion but state reality

6

A plan for a successful discharge from hospital to home: a further analysis of Roper's Activities of Living model

Alison Binnie

Introduction

Sending a patient home may be viewed by hospital staff as a satisfactory conclusion to an illness but for the patient and his family it may be only the beginning of a period of new challenges, new problems and major readjustment. It is possibly this difference in perspective which leads to some patients being sent out into the community with inadequate support or inadequately prepared to cope on their own. This chapter will open with a brief review of some of the research studies which have highlighted just how costly a poorly managed discharge from hospital can be in terms of human suffering and waste of health care resources. The problems identified in the research are not confined to the elderly alone, but there can be no doubt that the growing number of elderly people being sent back into the community, after surviving a period of critical illness in hospital, are particularly vulnerable to careless discharge planning.

The study of nursing care presented in this chapter concerns a severely disabled elderly woman at the point where she is about to be discharged from an acute surgical ward to the care of relatives, supported by the community services. At the time of this case, the ward nurses involved, used to a traditional style of practice, were just beginning to experiment with new patterns of work organisation and to consider new approaches to patient care. At this early stage in the ward's development, the discharge procedure was relatively unchanged. The account of a nursing-model-based discharge is therefore preceded by an outline of the ward's existing discharge procedure. A marked contrast will be noted between the rather limited and rigid traditional practice and the much more comprehensive and flexible model-based method.

The description of a model-based discharge, which forms the bulk of this chapter, incorporates a rationale for the choice of model, an outline of the theoretical basis of the model selected and finally, a short critique of the model in practice.

Research into problems associated with discharge from hospital

> Care must be planned, and planned before discharge, if it is to be continuous; very little was.

This was a disturbing conclusion drawn by Skeet (1970) as a result of her survey in which 533 patients were interviewed in hospital and then at home following discharge. She was seeking information on:

1 What discharged patients themselves see as their home care needs.
2 How these needs are being met.
3 The present hospital arrangements and existing community services for discharged hospital patients.

She found that many patients needed help with personal care immediately after returning home and that domestic work frequently presented a major problem. A coincidental finding was a great need for personal contact, particularly for the elderly:

> for almost two-thirds of the patients in the older age groups, interviewers had added a note such as 'very lonely', 'would like someone to chat to' or 'just sad'.

As well as attempting to identify and quantify some of the unmet needs of discharged patients, Skeet forcibly brings home to the reader how appalling and tragic the consequences of inadequate discharge planning can be by outlining the circumstances of eighteen of the 'worst instances of hardship' encountered during the study. The fact that fourteen of these eighteen patients were over the age of sixty-five supports the view that the elderly are particularly likely to suffer when there are failures in discharge planning.

A later survey, undertaken by two voluntary service organisers (Gay and Pitkeathley 1979), attempted to identify how a network of volunteers might be used to help meet the needs of people recently discharged from hospital. The account of interviews conducted during this survey shows vividly that unnecessary inconvenience and sometimes very real suffering were experienced by a number of the 257 patients and their families following the patients' discharge from hospital.

Unmet needs for care and inadequate preparation of discharged patients are evident in two other studies which involved interviewing recently discharged patients in their homes. Hockey (1968) was aiming to find out

> whether the contribution of the district nursing service to the care of discharged in-patients or current out-patients should be increased

and Roberts (1975) was attempting to devise tools which could be used to assess a patient's level of incapacity and his requirements for aftercare at home.

Whilst many social, environmental, financial and personal factors contribute to the hardships patients may experience when they go home from hospital, the studies mentioned above point to several areas where intervention by hospital nurses could prevent a great deal of suffering and reduce the often heavy burden carried by patients' families.

1 *Assessment of patients' needs and resources* The first step in any logical approach to planning appropriate care for a patient must be assessment of his need for care. In the case of a patient who is to be discharged from hospital, this must include collecting information about his home environment, assessment of his ability to care for himself in that environment and his family's ability to provide any support that is required.

Hockey (1968) found that, in many of the cases in her survey

> no one had assessed family need or resources, and the patients on interview revealed considerable anxiety and burden on their part.

In Skeet's (1970) survey, only 34% of female patients and 14% of male patients said they had been asked what their domestic arrangements would be when they left hospital and less than one-third of those aged sixty-six or more had been questioned on this topic. Similarly, in Roberts' (1975) study, respondents were asked whether anyone in hospital had discussed aftercare with them or with their relatives: only 18% definitely recalled any such discussion. Alarmingly, more than half the people with high Incapacity Scores (i.e. those most likely to need help with daily living activities) recalled no discussion of this nature.

2 *Provision of information and advice* As hospital nurses in these studies often failed to assess the needs of patients prior to discharge, it is perhaps not surprising that they also frequently sent them home with little or no appropriate advice or information.

Hockey (1968) found that, in her sample, 27% of patients requiring continuing medication or other treatment were ill-informed and anxious about their treatments. In Skeet's survey, 63% of the patients were discharged with drugs to take at home but of those, only 18% had received advice on dosage or possible side-effects.

Skeet also found there was great need for advice concerning activity: very few of the patients interviewed had been told how active they could be. What advice had been given by hospital staff was vague and ambiguous: "Don't do too much" or "Take care of yourself". Roberts' (1975) findings were similar;

> 42% of all respondents said they had received no advice at all . . . Relatively few people (15%) recalled any specific advice or instructions.

3 *Communication* Lack of pre-discharge assessment and information can be seen together as part of a larger problem of inadequate nurse-patient communication. Summarising her findings concerning 'Hospital Arrangements for Discharge of Patients', Skeet (1970) points this out;

> the greatest lack was one of communication . . . . In this study the patient needed information and advice about his illness and convalescence and staff needed information about the patient's home conditions and home care needs. Most of the maternity patients had this two-way communication; the majority of patients in other specialties did not.

An unpublished Scottish study (Clarke 1972), mentioned by Wilson-Barnett (1979) in her chapter discussing the stresses experienced by patients discharged from hospital, provides further examples of communication failures surrounding patients' return home from hospital. A quarter of the 376 patients in the study said they were not told what was wrong with them whilst in hospital and many complained of inadequate information. Nearly three-quarters of the patients were not asked if they needed help at home, although many were less active than before their admission.

Hospital nurses' communication with community staff is another area where there may be serious inadequacies. Hockey (1968) summarised the situation she found;

> communication between hospital and district nursing services was, on the whole, sparse and the paucity of information about patients, exchanged by verbal contact or written referral, was mutually regretted.

4 *Importance of discharge planning* Roberts' (1975) study included a small survey of ward sisters which aimed to assess their perceptions of the importance of discharge planning and the degree of priority they gave it in their own work. The findings are worrying;

> a majority . . . expressed a relatively low estimation of the importance of discharged patients' subsequent well-being as an element in their care, and most indicated that they regarded it as being entirely outside the proper range of nursing responsibilities.

The very few comments about discharge arrangements or about pre-discharge advice to patients or relatives that Roberts found when examining 156 sets of hospital records also seem to reflect the low priority hospital staff attached to discharge planning.

Gay and Pitkeathley (1979) mention one possible cause for hospital staff choosing to underestimate or ignore the problems their patients may have to face when they get home;

> there is no doubt that staff, particularly in acute hospitals, are under considerable pressure to discharge patients. 'They need the bed' is only too true. It seems, though, that their anxiety 'to keep the assembly line moving', as one patient put it, may lead the hospital staff to be over-optimistic in their assessment of what it would be like for the patient at home.

All of the studies mentioned in this section were carried out over five years ago. Since then, publication of the Nursing Times package containing practical guidelines on discharge planning (Skeet 1980), may have stimulated some ward nurses to review their discharge procedure, to give higher priority to preparation of patients going home and to improve communication with community services. Isolated, but nonetheless encouraging, reports now exist suggesting that at least some hospital nurses are beginning to take discharge planning seriously. For example, Barnett (1985) describes an attempt to link discharge planning and communication with community nurses to the development of the nursing process in hospital wards, and Gibb (1985) outlines a programme of self-medication for elderly patients in hospital as a preparation for going home.

Whilst there may have been some improvements in discharge planning in recent years, the annual reports of the Health Service Commissioner serve, in the absence of up-to-date research, to remind nurses that there is no room for complacency in this aspect of their work. Case histories revealing serious failures in discharge planning have featured with depressing regularity in the reports and in the most recent (Health Service Commissioner 1985), the Commissioner, in his introduction, mentions that

> complaints about the adequacy of the arrangements made for someone to leave hospital . . . appear frequently in the letters I receive.

Within the report itself, a whole section is devoted to complaints of this nature.

It is hoped that the case study presented in this chapter will demonstrate how a model of nursing can help nurses to approach a patient's discharge home in a realistic, thorough and organised manner, avoiding much of the distress that research studies suggest many patients experience when they leave hospital.

A surgical ward's discharge procedure

Early attempts to develop a systematic and individualised approach to nursing care in Ward A had involved the introduction of a relatively simple, structured assessment sheet in the nursing Kardex. This sheet included a section headed 'Home conditions and social arrangements'. The assessment sheet was usually completed within twenty-four hours of a patient's admission to the ward and some information would be recorded about home circumstances. This could subsequently be expanded as nurses got to know the patient and relatives better, but generally the amount of information was limited and there was rarely any obvious relationship between the nature of the information recorded and the kind of problems the patient might encounter on return home.

The ward doctors stated when they considered a patient to be medically fit for discharge, but they were willing to listen to a nursing view of the patient's readiness to manage at home and the final decision about a discharge date was usually negotiated, in the patient's presence, with his or her views being sought.

Patients were sometimes only given a few hours' notice of discharge, but this was usually following relatively minor surgery, when the patient had anticipated a short stay in hospital. In more complex situations, the discharge date was commonly agreed at least two or three days in advance.

There was a medical social worker who related specifically to the ward and who was thus well known to the nurses. He was involved when nurses were concerned about a patient's home circumstances and he often did follow-up visits if there were serious home problems.

Referral to the district nursing service was routine practice if a patient required continuing attention to a surgical wound and also quite often occurred when the patient being discharged was frail or in some way physically disabled following surgery. A standard form was sent with the patient for the district nurse, but the information provided was often sparse.

The front of the nursing record used in the ward incorporated a printed checklist for discharge arrangements. The nurses made little use of this, but they seemed to have a similar mental checklist relating to discharging patients and they could generally be relied upon to ensure that follow-up appointments were made, appropriate transport home arranged, drugs to take home provided and letters written to the General Practitioner and district nurse. The ward clerk played an important part in making these practical arrangements and she did record what had been done on the printed checklist.

During the week preceding the events described below, twenty-two patients were discharged from the ward. Whilst the practical arrangements just mentioned were made and recorded for all the patients, there was no indication in any of the nursing records that information or advice was either requested by the patient or provided by the staff. Although not recorded, some patients were witnessed receiving information prior to discharge, but this was usually in the form of routine instructions, for example, relating to removal of sutures, or a standard pattern of rest and exercise as following surgery for varicose veins. There was no reliable system for assessing patients' individual needs for information and advice or for assessing their ability to manage at home. What did occur was haphazard, unrecorded and often initiated by the patient.

Responsibility for discharge planning in the ward was vague. Making arrangements for sending patients home usually fell to the trained nurse in charge of a shift and the ward clerk. This worked adequately for the routine parts of the procedure, but for the more individual aspects, such as giving advice, teaching new skills, or seeing relatives, it was unreliable, particularly as so little of what was needed or what had already been provided was written down.

The following case history illustrates how vitally important these neglected elements of discharge planning can be and demonstrates how using a suitable model of nursing can ensure that they are systematically incorporated into the discharge procedure.

The patient

Emily Lawson was an Irish Catholic spinster of working class background. She had moved to England after the Second World War to find work and settled in Manchester where she had had several jobs either in factories or in domestic service. As she got older, she had taken part-time work and at the age of sixty-five had retired completely and lived off a state pension in a small council flat.

Emily had been the youngest of a large family, but having moved to England, she gradually lost touch with her brothers and sisters in Ireland and now they had all died. However, a married niece had moved to Manchester in 1970 and Emily had formed a close relationship with her and her family.

Emily was admitted to hospital in 1976 with a stroke. She went to stay with her niece, Margaret, for a month after this to convalesce and then, having made a complete recovery, returned to her own flat. A second stroke led to a similar pattern of events four years later, but by this time Margaret had moved to a small town near Oxford because her husband had changed his job. Emily had come to Oxfordshire to convalesce, but again she recovered sufficiently to return to an independent life in Manchester, coming to stay with Margaret two or three times a year for holidays.

In 1981 Emily had been diagnosed as having mild, late-onset diabetes mellitus. This had been controlled with oral hypoglycaemic agents and slight dietary modification—essentially just avoiding sugar and sweet foods.

At the beginning of 1984, Emily had come to stay with Margaret for a New Year holiday. She was now seventy-seven, her sight was failing as a result of cataracts and she was generally becoming rather frail. Margaret had invited her to stay on until the worst of the winter weather was over. During this time, Emily had developed a sore on her left foot. She could not remember when it had begun, but by the beginning of March she had wet gangrene on the first web space of the foot, with ascending cellulitis. The area was black, moist, smelly and painful.

Emily was admitted to hospital on 9th March and the following day she had a left below-knee amputation. Initially she made a good recovery: her diabetes was kept under control and her stump healed well. Then, two weeks after the operation, Emily had her third stroke. At first she was semi-comatose and had a dense left hemiplegia, but once again she began to recover and, by the end of April, although normal function had not returned to her left arm, she was fully alert, working hard with her physiotherapist and spending much of her time up in a wheelchair. Although she experienced understandable periods of frustration and regret, overall Emily accepted the loss of her limb and consequent disability as one of the unfortunate accompaniments of old age and she determined to make the best of her lot and to be as little trouble to others as possible.

Whilst not restored to independent function, and never likely to be, Miss Lawson was no longer critically ill and an acute hospital ward was neither the most congenial nor appropriate place for her to stay. The decision to experiment with a nursing model as a framework for discharge planning was taken at this stage. The starting point for this model-based discharge can thus be summarised as follows:

1. Miss Emily Lawson was medically fit for transfer out of an acute surgical setting.
2. She was psychologically reasonably well adjusted to her long-term disability.
3. She had been rehabilitated almost to her full physical potential, but she remained severely physically handicapped (i.e. she was wheelchair-dependent and required assistance with many basic activities of daily living).
4. She had extremely caring, highly motivated relatives who were willing to care for her in their home on a long-term basis.

The need for a nursing model

There was clearly potential in this situation for a successful discharge and long-term care for Miss Lawson in the community, amidst a family who were extremely fond of her. However, there were also many potential hazards and the existing discharge procedure in the ward was not adequate to ensure they would be avoided.

There was a need to work within a broader framework than the ward's checklist of routine arrangements. There needed to be a systematic and detailed assessment of the care Miss Lawson would need at home; careful planning and co-ordinated implementation of teaching and advice for the family; and effective liaison with community services. Miss Lawson needed to be aware of what could realistically be achieved and then helped to work towards these goals with an identified team of professionals who would provide consistent, co-ordinated support.

Pearson (1983) states that a conceptual model of nursing

> provides the unifying framework for an organised way of looking at nursing.

This was what was needed to guide nursing activity relating to Emily Lawson's discharge from hospital.

Selection of a nursing model

Pearson (1983), discussing the views of Orem and Roper on nursing concepts and theories, states that both theorists believe

> that a satisfactory model will describe nursing in any context: it will have meaning to nurses in all of the medical specialties, specialties arising from classification of age groups .... and specialties determined by the setting in which care is given.

Indeed, it can be argued that the validity of any model of nursing rests upon its being a reliable framework for practice in any nursing situation (Crow 1982). Whilst, as Crow points out, none of the nursing models described so far has been scientifically validated, neither has any one of them been conclusively dismissed as invalid in any particular nursing situation. Thus, whilst all the proposed nursing models "remain at the level of speculation" (Crow 1982), it would theoretically have been equally appropriate to select any one of them as a framework for organising Emily Lawson's discharge from hospital and subsequent care in the community. For example, Roy's stress adaptation model could have been used to identify adaptive and maladaptive behaviours within the physiological, self-concept, role function and interdependence modes. Then it would have been possible to plan nursing intervention aimed at manipulating Miss Lawsons's environment to produce healthy adaptation to the many stresses and changes confronting her (Roy 1980). Alternatively, Orem's model might have been used to identify self-care agents (the family and community services in this case) (Orem 1971).

At the end of a detailed analysis of four theoretical models of nursing (King's, Rogers',

Roy's and Orem's), McFarlane (1980) states that

the similarities are those of substance, and the differences are those of emphasis and semantics.

Thus, whilst any model could be used, these differences of emphasis and semantics can make one model more appropriate than another in certain circumstances. This was true in the case of Emily Lawson.

The model selected had to be built upon concepts that could easily be grasped by nurses trained in the traditional British system and to be expressed in language that would neither confuse nor deter them. Roy's self-concept, role function and interdependence modes would have been difficult for nurses with little or no training in the behavioural sciences to come to terms with in a short space of time. Equally, it would have been absurd to expect nurses taking their first tentative steps away from firmly established traditional, medical-model practice to grapple at once with Rogers' principles of reciprocy, syncrony, helicy and resonancy, in order to

promote symphonic interaction between man and the environment, to strengthen the coherence and integrity of the human field, and to direct and redirect patterning of the human and environment fields for realisation of maximum health potential! (Rogers 1972)

Whilst it may be possible to make valuable use of many of the American models of nursing after a suitably long period of background study, discussion and preparation of ward staff, the emphasis and particularly the semantics of the majority of the models rendered them totally inappropriate for presentation to staff in Ward A, at the stage of development it had reached when Emily Lawson was a patient there. The model described by Roper, Logan and Tierney (1980), on the other hand, seemed to have much to offer in spite of the constraints of the ward situation. As the only British model of nursing, it was the model of choice for use with nurses who had had no exposure to the semantics of American nursing theory: it is described in plain, everyday English. The core elements of the model, namely, a dependence-independence continuum, acti-

vities of living, and preventing, comforting and dependent components of nursing are relatively simple for the novice to grasp and apply in practice.

The main emphasis of the model, upon nursing activity aimed at helping people to cope with the practicalities of everyday living, was particularly appropriate for Emily Lawson. In addition, application of the model through a process involving assessment, planning, implementation and evaluation is now broadly familiar to most British nurses, at least in theory if not in practice, as opposed to processes described in some other models.

An outline of Roper's model of nursing

The model of nursing described by Roper *et al.* (1980) has been developed from a model of living and a model of nursing proposed by Roper (1976). The model of living focuses upon the individual person and presents the person involved in the business of living throughout his lifespan. In living, the person undertakes for himself, or requires help with, four groups of interrelated activities:

1 activities of living
2 preventing activities
3 comforting activities
4 seeking activities.

Performance of the activities of living involves the other three groups of activities, so that there can be preventing, comforting or seeking dimensions to the performance of any of the activities of living. Within the activities of living, throughout his lifespan, the person moves backwards and forwards along a dependence-independence continuum, his position on the continuum at any one time depending upon his stage of development, his state of health and his physical, psychological and social environment.

Roper *et al.* state that

since for most people illness is but an episode in life, it is useful to develop a similar way of thinking about the two processes—living and nursing.

Thus, their model of nursing focuses upon the patient, the subject of nursing, and places him on a lifespan, since nursing may be concerned with people at any stage between conception and death. The framework of activities of living and the dependence-independence continuum also appear in the model of nursing, since, as the authors state

> a very important aspect of nursing is assessing a patient's level of independence in all activities of living and judging in which direction, and by what amount, he should be assisted to move along his dependent/independent continua and what help he requires to meet the objectives set.

Components of nursing are also linked closely to the preventing, comforting and seeking activities which relate to the activities of living. Nursing is presented as having a preventing component (e.g. health education and preventing complications of illness and hospitalisation); a comforting component (e.g. maximising physical comfort, enhancing psychological and physical ability to cope with stress/illness); and a dependent component (related to seeking activities—when a patient is ill he may seek medical help and then require nursing; the dependent component of nursing is seen by Roper as medically prescribed).

Roper's model of nursing is applied in practice through the systematic, problem-oriented, 'process of nursing'. Activities of living provide a framework for nursing assessment. The dependent-independent continuum is a useful guide for identifying patients' problems and setting goals for care; and the preventing, comforting and dependent components of nursing, a helpful categorisation for nursing actions.

The model in action

When it became clear that Miss Emily Lawson was progressing beyond the stage where acute hospital care was appropriate for her, the possibility of sending her home to her family was discussed with the ward nurses. The complexity of the situation and the potential hazards of the discharge were emphasised. The proposal to try using a structured framework for planning the discharge was accepted. One newly qualified staff nurse, who felt she had established a good relationship with Miss Lawson and who was due to be on duty for five consecutive days prior to the discharge date, agreed to take special responsibility for assessing what was needed and for co-ordinating arrangements, under the ward sister's supervision.

Sister and staff nurse began by reviewing and writing a summary of the presenting situation (see Appendix I). They then worked out the broad goals for their discharge plan. These were also recorded at the beginning of the care plan and they were shared with Miss Lawson. Roper's model was now to be used to provide a framework for detailed assessment and for making plans which would achieve the goals that had been agreed.

The staff nurse had no previous experience of models of nursing, either in theory or in practice, so Roper's model was presented to her in a relatively simple way, emphasising the activities of living component and the dependent-independent continuum; and showing how, within this framework, it would be possible systematically to identify what Miss Lawson would be able to do for herself at home and where she would require assistance from others. Having established the areas of need, it would then be possible to talk with the family to find out whether they had the knowledge/skills/equipment/support they would need to help Emily compensate for her loss of independence.

The 'Assessment Data' recorded in the first column of the nursing care plan (see Appendix II) was collected over a period of two days by the staff nurse. She spent time observing and talking with Emily and she joined a 'family conference' attended by Margaret, her 17 year old daughter Caroline, the ward sister and the house surgeon, to discuss the practicalities of caring for Emily at home. (In retrospect, both sister and staff nurse thought it would have been appropriate to have brought Emily into the office for the family discussion, instead of following the traditional pattern of seeing patient and relatives separately.) The activities of living framework gave staff nurse a structure which helped her to focus upon important details in her nursing assessment and also helped her to record relevant information in a concise, logical way. Sister used the same framework at the family conference, guiding the discussion unobtrusively through the various activities of living, raising problem areas one at a time to explore with the family. This minimised the risk of confusion for the family and ensured that nothing was forgotten.

Staff nurse took notes of the new assessment data that emerged at the meeting and of the decisions that were reached about how care would be provided. She explained what had been suggested to Miss Lawson and confirmed that the plans met with her approval.

From the now fairly comprehensive assessment data it was possible for sister and staff nurse to identify problem areas with some precision and to write a plan of the nursing action required over the next few days to make sure problems were dealt with by the time Emily went home. An 'outcome' column was added to the care plan so that completed actions could be recorded. This addition to the record allowed other ward staff to see how the discharge arrangements were progressing and it avoided duplication and omission.

A column for writing a specific goal relating to each problem was not included in this plan. This was not because goal-setting as an essential and integral part of the nursing process was in any way questioned. It was rather because, in planning this kind of nursing activity, the desired outcome of nursing actions was either quite clear from the broad goals stated at the beginning of the plan or implied within the problem statement and/or nursing prescription.

Writing, in detail, every step of one's thinking may be a useful exercise for nurses just learning to plan their patients' care in a logical way. Recording, and sharing with the patient, precise specific goals that mark the steps in a gradual rehabilitative process, such as regaining independent mobility after a stroke, can be extremely helpful and worthwhile. However, writing an obvious statement clearly implied elsewhere, simply because one is bound by a rigid framework, can produce a clumsy, rather silly record that is laborious both to write and to read. For example, in Miss Lawson's plan, under 'assessment data' in relation to 'mobilising' it is noted that there are three steps leading out of Margaret's house at front and back and also that Emily likes going outdoors. This presents a 'problem'—ramps will have to be made if Emily is to be able to go out of the house in her wheelchair. A plan to make sure this work is carried out is written down. Including a 'goal' column in the plan would make this section read as follows:

Assessment	Problem	Goal	Nursing Plan	Outcome
Ground floor all on one level, but 3 steps to outside at front and back—Emily likes to be outdoors as much as possible.	Ramps needed to front and back doors.	Ramps will be made as soon as possible.	Contact medical social worker to make arrangements with Social Services Dept.	

Including goals like this in the plan would add nothing but unnecessary writing. The desired outcome, 'that ramps will be made', is implied in the plan as it stands and is encompassed by the initial broad goals (nos. 4 and 5, see p 90).

Thus whilst this particular care plan is not written by strictly adhering to the pattern Roper *et al.* (1981) have suggested, it is argued that this plan has still been devised by a logical process and includes the essential steps of problem-solving. Greater flexibility in recording the process of nursing, providing it demonstrates rational thought about individual patient problems, may help more nurses to see it as a method that can usefully and realistically be assimilated into busy practice.

The day before Miss Lawson went home, sister and staff nurse went through the care plan with her, considering their initial goals in relation to each activity of living and checking that all the arrangements and referrals they had planned had been arranged. Further evaluation of the effectiveness of their planning, in relation to Emily and the family coping at home, was not possible because hospital nurses do not have any follow-up contact with their patients. However, there was some feedback from the social worker after his home visits: he reported that everything was running very smoothly.

The value of using a model of nursing

The staff nurse who worked through Miss Lawson's discharge plan found the exercise an enlightening one. She said she had never realised how much there was to think about, or how easy it was to overlook small, but important things in a busy ward that discharged over a hundred patients a month. She found the model extremely helpful both as a framework for collecting and organising information that was relevant to Emily's care, and as a means of clarifying what she was aiming for—independence for Emily where it was feasible, an appropriate level of support where it was not.

It may be pointed out that if the model had been used earlier in Emily's care, some of the information staff nurse collected would already have been available and there would have been less last minute work to do. Similarly, it would also have been better to start the discharge planning and preparation of the family much earlier. Fortunately, because Margaret was so highly motivated and devoted to her aunt, she coped well with the situation, but many other relatives might have found it difficult to learn and to think about so much in the space of a few days.

Whilst the Roper, Logan and Tierney model undoubtedly provided a framework for discharge planning which was vastly superior to its predecessor in Ward A, and whilst it did seem to guide nursing activity at the end of Emily

Lawson's stay in hospital very effectively, a word of caution to nurses who may wish to undertake similar experiments in discharge planning must be added.

Within their model of living, Roper *et al.* (1980) have clearly tried to present a comprehensive view of the human individual, including social and psychological as well as biological aspects of living. Within each of the twelve activities of living which provide the framework for a systematic process of nursing, the authors recommend assessment of such areas as attitudes, knowledge, sociocultural factors, levels of independence and discomforts. However, although each of the activities may have psychological and social components, the named activity is essentially a physical activity of living (e.g. eating and drinking, mobilising, breathing etc.). Presentation of such a framework to present day nurses, who have inherited a strong bias towards physical aspects of care, could be misleading. To redress the balance of the traditional bias, model-makers of today would perhaps be wise to lay a rather clearer emphasis, within the basic structure of their models, upon the holistic nature of the human individual. For example, inclusion of the predominantly mental activities of 'being' or 'suffering' in the Roper *et al.* framework would stress the need for nurses to concern themselves with such neglected areas as self-concept, body-image, self-esteem, personal values, motivation, religious faith, anxiety, fear, mutilation, insecurity, loss, grief and pain. Whilst Roper *et al.* do not intend to ignore these areas of human experience, it may be suggested that, in a model for present day nursing, they need to be given a much more prominent place.

Emily Lawson's problems in preparing to adapt to life in the community did appear to be largely of a practical nature. However, with the use of a model which more obviously led the nurses to focus on non-physical aspects of living, other problems could have emerged.

Conclusion

The use of a model of nursing to manage Emily Lawson's complicated discharge from hospital enabled her nurses to provide detailed and highly individualised nursing support. It provided a valuable learning experience for a junior staff nurse, in particular, helping her to see nursing in a broader perspective than the traditional process of completing routine tasks. The Roper, Logan and Tierney model, chosen to guide this patient's discharge from hospital, proved to be intelligible and acceptable to nurses who had no previous exposure to modern nursing theory. In this particular case, the model appears to have led to a suitably comprehensive nursing assessment and plan of care. It is likely that it may be equally valuable for planning the discharge from hospital of a great many other disabled, elderly patients, provided that nurses guard against a superficial appreciation of the model which could easily lead to neglect of the psychosocial elements of nursing care.

References

Barnett D 1985 The information exchange. *Nursing Times*, 81, 9: 27–29.

Clarke MO 1972 An Aspect of Communication in the Health Service, Unpublished Research Report. *Cited in*: Wilson-Barnett, J. *Stress in hospitals*. Churchill Livingstone, Edinburgh.

Crow R 1982 Frontiers of nursing in the twenty-first century: development of models and theories on the concept of nursing, *Journal of Advanced Nursing*, 7: 111–116.

Gay & Pitkeathley 1979 *When I went home, A study of patients discharged from hospital.* King Edward's Fund, London.

Gibb S 1985 "The yellow one is my water pill". *Nursing Times*, 81, 9: 29–30.

Health Service Commissioner 1985 *Annual Report for 1984–1985.* HMSO, London.

Hockey L 1968 *Care in the balance: a study of collaboration between hospital and community services.* Queens Institute of District Nursing.

King IM 1971 *Towards a theory for nursing.* John Wiley, New York.

McFarlane EA 1980 Nursing theory: the comparison of four theoretical proposals. *Journal of Advanced Nursing*, 5: 3–19.

Orem DE 1971 *Nursing: concepts of practice.* McGraw-Hill, New York.

Pearson A 1983 *The clinical nursing unit.* Heinemann Medical Books, London.

Roberts I 1975 *Discharged from hospital.* Royal College of Nursing Research Project, Series 2 No. 6. RCN, London.

Rogers ME 1972 *An introduction to a theoretical basis of nursing.* F A Davis Company, Philadelphia.

Roper N 1976 A model for nursing and nursology. *Journal of Advanced Nursing*, 1: 219–227.

Roper N, Logan W & Tierney AJ 1980 *The elements of nursing.* Churchill Livingstone, Edinburgh.

Roper N, Logan W & Tierney AJ 1981 *Learning to use the process of nursing.* Churchill Livingstone, Edinburgh.

Roy C 1980 The Roy Adaptation Model. In Riehl JP & Roy C (Eds) *Conceptual models for nursing practice*, 2nd Ed. Appleton-Century-Crofts, Norwalk.

Skeet M 1970 *Home from hospital.* Dan Mason Nursing Research Committee of the Florence Nightingale Memorial Committee of Great Britain & Northern Ireland.

Skeet M 1980 *Discharge procedures, practical guidelines for nurses.* Macmillan, London.

Wilson-Barnett J 1979 *Stress in hospital—patients' psychological reactions to illness and health care.* Churchill Livingstone, Edinburgh.

Appendix I

Date	Summary of presenting situation	Broad goals for discharge planning	Signature
3.4.84	Miss Lawson: —is medically fit for transfer out of an acute, surgical setting. —is psychologically reasonably well adjusted to her long-term disability. —has been rehabilitated almost to her full physical potential. —but she remains severely physically handicapped (i.e. is wheelchair-dependent & requires assistance with many basic activities of daily living). —has extremely caring, highly motivated relatives who are willing to care for her in their home on a long-term basis.	1) Emily will retain maximum independence within the limits of her severe disability. 2) Measures will be taken to prevent complications that could occur as a result of her disabilities. 3) Emily and her family will acquire the skills and knowledge needed to achieve the above (1 & 2) before Emily leaves hospital. 4) Equipment required to achieve goals 1) and 2) will be available to the family at the time of discharge. 5) Referrals will be made to ensure that the family have access to appropriate practical support and professional advice in the community.	

Unit No. 123456	Consultant:	Surname: LAWSON
		Forename(s): Emily

Appendix II

	ASSESSMENT DATA	PROBLEM	NURSING PLAN	OUTCOME
Date 4.4.84.				
Maintaining a safe environment	Risk factors—visual impairment & severely limited mobility. But Emily is aware of her limitations & calls for assistance before attempting any potentially hazardous acitivity. Familiar with geography of niece's house.			
Communicating	Good relationship with niece & family. Used to being a guest in their home. Has expressed some sadness at giving up an independent home & dislikes 'being a trouble to others', but is making appropriate psychological adjustment—'you have to accept these things at my age'. 'I've always been happy at Margaret's, they're very good to me'.			
	Impaired vision due to cataracts—referral to eye specialist made—appointment in 3 months. Is able to recognise people at 2–3 feet. Needs food, drink etc. placing nearby—family aware & able to compensate appropriately.	Will need transport to eye Clinic	Ward clerk to arrange	
	Slightly impaired speech following stoke and no dentures and strong Irish accent makes her difficult to understand at times—Irish family have less difficulty than nurses. Mentally alert, able to participate in group interaction. Has retained warm sense of humour.	Wants new dentures	(see under Eating & Drinking)	
Breathing	No discomforts/difficulties with breathing. Gave up smoking after first stroke.			
Eating and Drinking	Has always been slim. Currently thin, but not seriously undernourished. Has been eating 3 meals a day for last week—esp. likes fish, chicken, brown bread & butter. Willingly drinks $1\frac{1}{2}$–2 litres fluid/day—likes weak tea & diabetic lemon juice.			
Unit No. 123456	Consultant:		Surname: Lawson	Forename(s): Emily

Date 4.4.84.	ASSESSMENT DATA	PROBLEM	NURSING PLAN	OUTCOME
Eating and Drinking (continued)	Mild diabetic. Takes Glibenclamide 5 mg × 2 daily and avoids sweet foods.	Family unclear about diet—would like more information	Arrange for Margaret & Caroline to see dietitian	Seen by dietitian 6.4 Written information provided. Now feels confident
	Dentures have become too big for gums—uncomfortable to wear—restricts eating—would like new set.	Needs new dentures	Margaret to contact local dentist	
	Loss of fine control of left hand due to stroke makes eating difficult. Has been managing to feed herself in hospital using modified utensils & non-slip plate mat. Family aware that food needs to be cut up finely for her—they have been present at hospital meal times.	Will need special eating utensils at home so she can continue to feed independently	Ask social worker about transport Ask Occupational Therapist to liaise with community OT service	Voluntary services will help. Margaret given phone number Community OT will visit day after discharge
Eliminating	Continent of urine & faeces during daytime, provided she can call for assistance. Needs help from one person to transfer from chair or bed to commode. Margaret's downstairs toilet probably too small for wheelchair and space limited for transfer manoeuvre.	(see Mobilising) Feasibility of using downstairs toilet during daytime needs assessment	Refer to OT	
	Margaret does not possess a commode.	Needs commode before discharge	Contact Red Cross re loan of commode	Red Cross will deliver commode 7.4.84
	Emily is occasionally incontinent at night—usually through not calling for help in time—controlled in hospital by night nurse getting her up to commode at 10 pm before settling & again at 4 am, i.e. not more than 6 hour gap. Margaret usually goes to bed at midnight & wakes early am—prepared to get up to attend to Emily. Would like some incontinence drawsheets 'just in case'. Has automatic washing machine—could cope with occasional 'accident'. Margaret's bedroom is upstairs, Emily to sleep downstairs.	Preventable nocturnal urinary incontinence Supply of absorbent drawsheets needed Emily needs to be able to call for assistance	Margaret to help Emily to commode at midnight and 6 am Discuss with District Nurse Margaret has handbell for daytime. Will borrow 'baby alarm' intercom from married daughter for night time	D N phoned—will visit with sheets on 9.4.84 pm

		Problem		Prescribed
	Emily was prone to constipation in hospital—likely to continue due to immobility. Controlled on 2 tbs bran on cereal am. Wholemeal bread and 10 ml Normacol granules at night—bowels open every one or two days.	Potential constipation	Margaret to continue bran and brown bread. Needs Normacol TTO To inform District Nurse if bowels not open for four days	
Personal Cleansing and Dressing	Emily can wash her face, hand, front of her trunk and pelvic region using her right hand, if provided with necessary equipment. She cannot wash her back, her bottom, or her right foot—two people needed to wash bottom—one to support her, one to wash, unless washed in bed.	Needs help with washing	Margaret and Caroline to come to hospital Sat & Sun mornings to help Emily wash	Managed well. Emily pleased. Confident they will cope at home
	Pressure areas—unable to turn herself in bed—position changed 3 hourly by nurses—not possible at home during night. Small (1 cm diameter) superficial sacral sore developed since Emily has been spending long periods in wheelchair. Risk of pressure sores and principles of prevention understood by Margaret and Caroline—will inspect skin daily.	Risk of pressure sores developing at night	Ask District Nurse to supply ripple mattress	DN will supply on 9.4.84
		Risk of non-healing or further development of sacral pressure sore	Ask OT to provide battery operated ripple cushion and instruct family in use	Provided 7.4.84 Family understand charging and maintenance.
	Right foot—chiropodist attended a week ago—skin and nails currently in good condition, but diabetic + recent gangrene → amputation. Unable to see her own foot clearly or to care for skin and nails.	High risk of serious infection if skin on right foot is damaged	Margaret to wash and inspect foot 2 or 3 times weekly. To report any skin lesion to District Nurse. To arrange monthly chiropody visit to home (will contact health centre)	
	Hyperactivity of left arm makes dressing difficult. Cannot manage any garment independently, but will co-operate and participate. Independence may increase if control of arm improves. Aware of importance of soft comfortable shoe	Needs help with dressing.	Margaret and Caroline to help Emily dress in hospital on Sat & Sun. To encourage independence if arm improves with time	Successful. All feel confident to manage at home

Unit No. 123456 Consultant: Surname: Lawson Forename(s): Emily

Date 4.4.84.	ASSESSMENT DATA	PROBLEM	NURSING PLAN	OUTCOME
Mobilising	Left below knee amputation. Recent R CVA—power returned to left arm, but control very limited—frequent involuntary movements. Cannot balance in standing position. Can propel wheelchair a few feet using right arm, but poor vision makes this inadvisable unless 2nd person present—Emily aware of risks.	Needs assistance: 1) to transfer from bed to chair and from bed/chair to commode, 2) to propel wheelchair	Margaret and Caroline to learn transfer technique from physio—Thurs and Fri at 3 pm. To practise under supervision of nurses over weekend	8.4.84 Both have mastered technique— able to protect themselves and move Emily comfortably
	Family are currently having downstairs of house extended so Emily can have what was the living room as her own room. Ground floor all on one level, but 3 steps to outside at front and back—Emily likes to be outdoors as much as possible.	Ramps needed to front and back doors	Contact medical social worker to make arrangments with Social Services Dept	Ramps can be made, but will be several weeks before they are done.
	Needs ambulance to take her home.	Ambulance to be booked	Ward clerk to arrange	Booked for 9.4.84.am Family informed
Working and Playing	Emily receives a state pension—she has asked Margaret to accept this as a contribution to 'her keep'. Building work to house, though seen as a long term investment, is a major financial burden at present.	Financial strain for family as a result of building work necessary to accommodate Emily.	Contact medical social worker to investigate 1) Eligibility for grant for building work 2) Eligibility for attendance allowance 3) Possibility of residential holiday relief care in summer	Social worker will make home visit on 12.4.84 and will follow up
	There will be some restriction of family leisure activities as a result of caring for Emily. Margaret doesn't go out a lot—Women's Institute meetings, occasional bingo & shopping—can arrange for Caroline or husband (Bill) to be at home then. Only real problem to Margaret is the family summer holiday. Emily's activities very limited. Likes 'to be with people'—enjoys being in the heart of the family, takes great interest in their activities. Likes listening to the radio—has her own transistor. Likes being out of doors (see under Mobilising).	Restriction to family leisure activities because Emily cannot be left alone		
	Used to go to Catholic Church to mass about once a month in Manchester. No Catholic Church near Margaret's home.	Unable to maintain usual church attendance	Margaret will ask priest to visit regularly	

Expressing Sexuality	Previous periods of dependence & long episodes of hospitalisation have enabled her to overcome embarrassment at needing help with intimate procedures—washing, toiletting etc. Now seems relatively comfortable accepting this kind of help from female relatives. Maintains healthy concern about her appearance—interest in what she wears etc.	
Sleeping	Has always slept soundly. Never takes sedatives. Had no problems sleeping in hospital. Like to settle early—about 10 pm & wakes about 6 am. Likes 2 pillows. Likes to rest on bed for an hour after lunch.	Margaret will maintain usual pattern at home
Dying	Realistic attitude to her old age. Accepts inevitability of death. During early days of rehabilitation, felt the effort involved wasn't worthwhile, 'I wish I could have just died on the table' 'It doesn't seem worth all the bother when you're my age'. Now has a more positive attitude. Interested in living and sharing family life.	

Unit No. 123456   Consultant: Surname: Lawson   Forename(s): Emily

7

Dying: an examination of the Deficit model

Ann Faulkner

Dying, although inevitable for all of us, tends to be a taboo subject, not mentioned when one is well, and perhaps avoided when a person is known to be dying. As a consequence the bereaved are often also avoided because appropriate words of comfort cannot be found.

This reticence about death continues in the health professions. Brewin (1977) talks of 'the pretence and insincerity of false optimism', while Mackintosh (1977), who studied patients on a cancer ward, suggested that they did not wish to know their diagnosis or prognosis. Perhaps a more important finding here was that those patients who *did* wish to know had great difficulty in gaining an honest picture of their future.

That dying is avoided as a subject is hardly surprising since it represents leaving the known world for the unknown. Kubler-Ross (1975) describes death as 'the final stage of growth' while Roper *et al.* (1980) describe it as an activity of living. Such descriptions foster the Christian ethic of a 'hereafter'. Other beliefs about what happens after death include reincarnation, and atheism, which sees death as a total end of an individual's existence.

It might be thought that the elderly would be more prepared to die than younger people. The elderly may have more experience of death as relatives and friends die before them, but may have no wish to join them. Death can seem fearful at any age, especially to those with little or no religious belief (Brink 1979), and even those elderly people with little apparent quality of life may still have goals to reach and ambitions to fulfil.

One commonly held theory which might lead to a belief that the elderly are prepared to die is that of 'disengagement'. It is argued that the elderly set about disengaging from society. The counter argument is that society neglects to include the elderly in community activities. The 'generation gap' is not synonymous with a death wish on the part of the elderly who may feel that they are no longer useful to society.

Many nurses encounter death for the first time in hospital (Simpson 1975). They may be less upset if the dying patient is elderly since there is still a belief that those who have achieved 'three score years and ten' have had their allotted time. However, even with the elderly, death may be seen as a failure if the object of care is cure.

Elements of the Deficit nursing model

Faulkner (1985) describes nursing as 'a function which responds to an individual's reactions to deficits in his normal life pattern'. This approach uses psychological theory as a basis, particularly that of Maslow (1954) and Rogers (1961). It could be argued that there is nothing new in such an approach since the nursing process is based on meeting needs and helping patients achieve their potential. In fact the difference in approach is that care is considered from the patient's perspective, thus avoiding an over-simplification of theories which were formulated to explain normal personality development.

Maslow (1954) explained personality development in terms of a hierarchy of needs. He argued that if basic physiological needs for food, air and water were not met, higher order needs would become unimportant. In nursing process terms, such reasoning may be interpreted to mean that physical problems are always more important than social or psychological needs (Gingell 1985).

This is an over-simplification, and Faulkner points out that Maslow's theory was not designed to order priorities for patients, but to explain personality development in humans. Many people who are ill do not have severe deficits in basic physiological functioning. If they do, then obviously life-saving measures must be taken. If they do not, then the patients' perception of priorities must be considered.

Rogers' theory is similar. The concept of meeting potential is considered in the light of patients who have deficits due to ill-health which will *affect* their ability to maintain, or work towards, their potential. Such an approach allows for full potential to be reached within the physical limitations of a patient.

This psychological underpinning of the nursing process approach to care differs from that of authors such as Roper (1980) and Orem (1971) which are mainly concerned with an individual's ability to continue with self care. The deficit model is rather more concerned with an individual's reaction to deficits, diagnosis, prognosis and treatment and the effect this will have on his normal functioning.

It is not unusual for nursing theorists to use other disciplines as a foundation for nursing. The Roper model, for example, draws from physiological, psychological and sociological theory in order to set the parameters for nursing care. What is not clear is the particular way in which such theories are used except in their relevance to the normal activities of daily living. Differences in the use of psychological theories may seem subtle but are in fact profound. In Roper's model, for example, much depends on an individual's ability to function normally. Orem is concerned with encouraging self care. Both these theorists appear to use a system which militates against the 'sick role' as described by Parsons (1966), in that nursing is geared towards goals of activities of daily living being resumed or self care being achieved. By these criteria, dying could be seen as failure, though Roper separates it from the continuum of self care by designating death as a separate activity of living.

One point arising from this is the suitability of any model for all situations. Certainly a model based on activities of living will have limitations in many areas. In hospital for instance, many activities of daily living are inappropriate. These include expressions of personality by choice of clothes and jewellery, expressions of sexuality, and the following of work and leisure pursuits. Even eating as a social act may be curtailed. The major activities of daily living which remain are mainly biological and concerned with survival. That is, no matter how different an environment the patient finds himself in, he will still need to breathe, eat, drink, eliminate and keep clean. From this it may be seen that the emphasis in Roper's model is biological.

It may be that nurses should be prepared to use models in an eclectic way. If, for example, it is agreed that Roper's model has a strong biological basis and that the deficit model has a strong psychological basis, it can be seen that each will have particular applications. It is argued here that dying is not an activity of living but an ending of life on earth. As such it is best dealt with by using a model strong on psychological theory, for although physical deterioration will occur, the problems paramount will be those concerned with accepting (or rejecting) the imminence of death. The deficit model, with its emphasis on patient perception, allows for the individual who will not get well and may in fact deteriorate. This is important in the care of the dying patient since it allows for an honest approach to death which should not be associated with failure because the individual may not maintain an ability to care for himself.

Many theorists discuss nursing the dying patient. Henderson (1960) talks of helping a patient to a 'dignified death', while Roper *et al.* (1980) also talk of death with dignity. The literature on the nursing process, however, generally suggests setting goals for improvement using a problem-solving approach. Using patients' deficits as a starting point with a problem *identification* approach, it can be seen that it is not mandatory to solve all problems. With the dying patient, unless death is seen as the solution to his problems, there will be many insoluble problems, especially if goals are seen to be only possible in a positive direction. In the deficit model, patients with degenerative conditions and those who are dying may have goals set in a negative direction if improvement is not possible. By careful and regular assessment, each patient will be encouraged to reach his potential at any time, even though it may be less than previously.

Briefly, this approach is geared to each patient achieving the best possible quality of life each day. It will not always be successful immediately. The dying patient who has not accepted his prognosis may have equal difficulty in accepting increasing limitations on his life. This will be a problem for nursing staff but should not deter them from the goal of helping the patient reach a peaceful death, having achieved as much as possible on each day prior to the death.

One problem which may be anticipated in the deficit model is that it may not be immediately obvious that care is based on the patient's strengths as well as his deficits. Another way of putting this is that the patient will be encouraged to continue activities as he is able, while accepting that other activities may need to be curtailed. In this respect, assessment is a vital step in the nursing process. Deficits in knowledge should be identified along with the patient's readiness to accept the prognosis. Similar assessment should be made for physical, social and other psychological deficits which represent problems for the patient.

Individuals' reactions to deficits will vary. Many elderly people suffer from multiple pathology and may have lived with chronic illness for years. Although no assumptions may be made without assessment, it is possible that a patient may have developed mechanisms to cope with physical disability. Dying represents a different problem as the patient faces the unknown. This and other new problems arising as a result of terminal illness mean that psychological and social deficits may be more threatening to the patient than the physical problems with which he is familiar.

As a result of assessment, problems may be categorised into three groups as follows:

1   Problems directly related to the current illness

2   Problems not related to the current illness, but pertinent

3   Problems totally separate from the current illness.

In each category, problems may be subdivided into those which are actual and those which are potential. Problems should be further categorised in terms of their priority to the patient.

One argument against goals that move in a negative direction is that nurses may 'give up' and cease to make an effort with dying patients. The patients are then confined to bed and uselessness far earlier than is necessary. However, accurate and ongoing assessment should prevent this happening and actually diminish the patients' feelings of hopelessness.

An example of this is mobility. A patient who is made to sit out of bed in a chair to prevent him becoming bedfast, but who is not assessed to see what he might realistically achieve, may feel totally demoralised if he is tired after a short time. In trying to reach the goal of sitting out of bed for a proportion of each day, he may become exhausted but fail to complain. He may dread getting out of bed as his exhaustion builds up and when he finally *has* to stay in bed, he feels a failure.

In the deficit model, the patient's perspective is important. He should feel free to express his tiredness, and occasional days in bed may occur. There will in this instance be a less sharp distinction between getting up and staying in bed than when the patient feels duty bound to get up, to show that he is aiming for positive goals. In the latter case, not only will staying in bed equate with failure but it will also be identified with the final stage of illness.

The deficit model centres on the patient and his perception of his problems using the stages of the nursing process. Thus it concentrates on care of the patient as an individual with a background, a family and social commitments. As such, relatives are seen as an important component in patient care and they also have their own needs. This model and its applicability to the care of the dying elderly patient is best illustrated with a case study.

History

Mrs. Pat Davis was 78 years old, living with her husband George, who was 80 years old. Both had been very active, enjoying retirement since George gave up his manual work fifteen years ago. Mrs. Davis had devoted her life to her husband and child, occasionally taking a part-time cleaning job in someone's home to earn money for luxuries. She had been the 'strong' partner in that she had dealt with the decisions and crises of family life, shielding her husband from worries as far as possible.

Mrs. Davis was admitted to a medical ward with a diagnosis of carcinoma of the stomach with suspected metastatic spread. A laparotomy was performed and the carcinoma found to be inoperable. Mrs. Davis's condition was seen to be terminal although the consultant told her that he had 'sorted out a twist of bowel' and wanted her to concentrate on getting well. Mr. Davis was told that his wife's outlook was poor and that he should not expect her to be well enough to return home before she died. He agreed that his wife should not be told of the severity of her condition.

A care plan based on the Deficit model

The assessment of Mrs. Davis was carried out in two stages as suggested by McFarlane and Castledine (1982). On admission, the nurse was concerned to make Mrs. Davis feel comfortable, to find out her basic background and what she believed about her illness. In-depth assessment was carried out three days after the operation when the effects of the anaesthesia had worn off and the patient was feeling comfortable enough to talk to the nurse.

A modified version of the assessment form developed by Tait *et al.* (1982) was used by the nurse who had learned the necessary communication skills to elicit the problems and deficits as perceived by the patient. The initial assessment is shown in Figure 7.1, p 100.

From this initial assessment and from physical assessment and observations, Mrs. Davis' problems and deficits were identified. An interview with Mr. Davis elicited the information that his wife's fears for his welfare were well founded. He confessed that he had not been involved in shopping, cooking or cleaning, seeing them as 'women's work'. While his wife was in hospital his main diet consisted of baked beans and sausages or meals from the local 'carry out'.

Mr. Davis was, however, unperturbed by his state. He was more concerned for his wife, knowing that she might well have difficulties in adapting to a more dependent role as her condition deteriorated. He had not thought to discuss matters with his son. 'Pat writes all the letters – I didn't think'. However, on the nurse's suggestion, he agreed to telephone his son and share his concerns.

Problems and priorities

Of the key problems listed on p.101, it can be seen that they are all directly related to the patient's current illness. Mrs. Davis obviously led a full and happy life before her illness, and although she would like to have seen more of her son and his family, she had no major problems which affected her physical or mental health. It is however important to assess home background and support networks since problems may exist which affect a patient's reaction to illness or treatment.

Post-operatively, Mrs. Davis had a number of physical problems. Assessment on the scale devised by Norton *et al.* (1975) put her at risk of pressure sores. She had nutritional problems since her appetite was poor, and a problem of constipation. Her wound leaked and showed little sign of healing. Further, the leakage was offensive, causing embarrassment to her. Although she was able to walk with help, reduced mobility was seen to be a potential problem. Other potential problems were identified as pain and reduced energy.

Psychological problems were those identified in Figure 7.1. One potential problem was increased anxiety in the absence of an adequate

Fig. 7.1 Initial assessment of Mrs. Davis

1   **Demographic**
   Date of admission   6.5.85   **Hospital No.**   94699
   Name   Pat DAVIS   **Date of birth**   7.2.1907
   Name patient likes to be called   Mrs Davis
   Marital status   Married   **Occupation**   Retired
   Address   1 Manor Row
                 Dalvenie Road
                 Axminster
                 Devon
   Tel. no.   1591
   Next of kin   Mr George Davis   **Relationship**   Husband
   Occupation   Retired Builders Labourer
   Address   S/A

   Tel. No.   As above
   G.P.   Dr Scott
   Address   The Surgery, Axminster
   Tel. No.   5079
   Religion   C/E   **Importance of Religion**   Regular Church attender. Involved in Church affairs
      e.g. Mothers' Union
   Reason for admission   'prolonged stomach trouble' (Ca. Stomach)
   Previous hospitalisation with reasons   2 years ago had operation to remove 'wart' from face
   Current medication with dosage   Milk of magnesia before meals
   Others living in patient's home   Husband

2   **Current Disease**

   Patient's understanding of disease   Sees illness as 'upset stomach' which made her sick. Seems doubtful
   of doctor's 'twisted bowel' explanation but did not ask for alternative explanation
   Patient's understanding of present treatment (if known)   Thinks the operation may have
   'cleared a blockage' but sounds unconvinced
   Patient's previous experiences which might affect current perceptions   Mother and sister died
   of cancer. Doesn't know site of Ca. in Mother. Sister had cancer of ovaries (died at 52 years)
   Recent stressful events or chronic difficulties   Only son and grandchildren (all married) live some
   distance away. Lack of contact worries her.

3   **Key Relationships.**

   Patient's perception of partner in terms of expected support
   a   **Practical**   Husband not a practical man – can't cook or clean
   b   **Emotional**   Very supportive

   Patient's perception of family in terms of expected support
   a   **Practical**   Too far away to help
   b   **Emotional**   Will telephone and write. 'They do care'

   Patient's perception of friends in terms of expected support
   a   **Practical**   Neighbours very helpful. Will shop, etc.
   b   **Emotional**   No really close friends

   Patient's responsibilities to partner, family and friends
   a   **Partner**   'Looking after him takes all my time'
   b   **Family**   No responsibilities
   c   **Friends**   Church activities e.g. flowers, brass, etc.

Fig. 7.1 (continued)

4   Social

Patient's problems with:
a   **Housing**   None. Own bungalow
b   **Household responsibilities**   Very tired and 'out of sorts'
c   **Work**   Chores and church work have suffered
d   **Finance**   Income 'adequate' but not much to spare

Patient's normal leisure activities (include health hazards e.g. smoking, alcohol consumption):
Likes whist drives and driving in countryside. Drinks home-made wine regularly. This upsets stomach lately
so has 'cut down'. Takes 1–2 glasses each evening.

5   Psychological
Patient's reaction to current disease

Weight change: **Present**   9st 2lbs
                       Previous   11st 0lbs
                       Time span   4 months
Appetite change: **Present**   Poor – doesn't enjoy food
                       Previous   Good
                       Time span   3 months
Sleep change: **Present**   Sleeps well but early waking
                       Previous   Used to sleep until 7.30 am
                       Time span   'a few weeks'

Signs of anxiety. Specify: Appears anxious about diagnosis and about husband's ability to look after
   himself.
Signs of depression. Specify: No obvious signs of depression. Early waking but no weepiness. Can be
   distracted from anxiety about diagnosis.

6   Key problems
   1. Lack of information about diagnosis and prognosis.
   2. Unwillingness to discuss diagnosis and prognosis.
   3. Anxiety about husband's ability to cope (could be exacerbated if prognosis accepted).
   4. Poor appetite.
   5. Early waking. Her worries are worse at this time of day.

explanation for her lack of progress after operation. However, since Mrs. Davis's prognosis was
poor, other problems could be expected which
were associated with dying. No assumptions
could be made about the nature of these problems, which would be identified at assessment.

Once problems are identified, it is tempting to
give priority to physical problems. However,
some research suggests that stress may contribute
to physical illness (Cooper 1983), so psychological
problems may need to be given priority when
planning patient care. In fact, in the elderly dying
patient, no assumptions may be made about the
individual's acceptance of her own mortality.

Except in an emergency, priorities in terms of
problems and plans for care should be set from
the patient's perception of their importance. In
assessing Mrs. Davis the nurse listed as problems
lack of information and unwillingness on the
patient's part to discuss diagnosis and prognosis.
This raises questions as to whether the problem is
the patient's or the nurse's (Faulkner 1985). The
nurse had picked up cues from the patient
suggesting that there was uncertainty of belief.
Even so, the timing for giving information should
be linked to the patient's expressed needs. Many
dying patients actually deny the reality of their
prognosis.

For a nurse who believes that patients should accept the fact of their impending death, the denying patient may pose a problem. What needs to be made clear however is that the problem is the nurse's, not the patient's. Nurses may have learned of the five stages of dying (Kubler-Ross 1973), which are denial, anger, bargaining, depression and acceptance. They may feel that there is a need to plan goals towards acceptance. In fact, by remembering that care should be planned to reduce deficits and meet patients' needs, it becomes easier for a nurse to accept that some patients *need* to deny impending death.

Priorities for care for Mrs. Davis were set according to her perception of her condition and the nurse's knowledge of the risks involved. Mrs. Davis understood the priority of preventive care which was aimed at preserving the integrity of her skin and her personal hygiene. Priority was also given to her mental state. This included allocating time to allow her to talk through her concerns and to increase her knowledge when she felt ready to discuss the diagnosis and prognosis.

In terms of deficits in mobility and appetite, goals were not set for improvement. Rather, it was agreed that Mrs. Davis would get up and walk to the toilet if she felt able, but could have a commode if she preferred. This flexibility reduced the stress which might have been caused by unrealistic expectations. Similarly with diet, Mrs. Davis was not pressured to eat if she did not want to, but agreed to take milky drinks which she could tolerate. Figure 7.2 (p 103) shows part of a care plan for Mrs. Davis.

Nursing care

Initially, caring for Mrs. Davis was relatively simple. She had rationalised her weak condition in terms of the aftermath of major surgery. She appeared to suffer no pain and was quiet and cooperative. She suffered suppositories for her constipation without complaint, managed to walk with help to the toilet and dealt with her perceived problem of odour from her wound with the liberal use of lavender water.

The nurses who cared for Mrs. Davis described her as quiet and pleasant. It was therefore a shock to the nurse, who was helping her out of bed one day, to be pushed aside and hear, 'Oh, go away – I'm not a child – I want to manage on my own!' The nurse, surprised by the anger, tried to remonstrate, only to suffer a further outburst followed by tears. Sitting down by Mrs. Davis, she said, 'You seem very angry, tell me about it.' This open approach allowed Mrs. Davis to air her concerns and the nurse to make detailed assessment of the psychological problems which had been 'bottled up'. It soon became clear that Mrs. Davis was aware that she was not improving and was worried about both her own and her husband's future. Further, her spiritual beliefs were wavering in the face of her problems.

It was obvious that for Mrs. Davis the stage of denial was over but that there were deficits in her knowledge, concern about the future and a lessening of comfort from religion. Because she was able to air these concerns, the stage of anger was relatively short-lived. Anger may be sustained if a patient feels that she cannot talk to, or get the truth from, members of the health care team.

In eliciting Mrs. Davis's concerns, the nurse felt constrained by Mr. Davis's request that his wife should not know the truth. Such collusion is common in terminal illness. It may be that a partner wishes to protect a loved one or it may be that he has fears of his own in facing an unpleasant reality. The nurse had the following conversation with Mr. Davis:

Nurse: Mr Davis, your wife knows that she is not getting better. I think she will soon want to talk about her future.
Mr. Davis: Don't tell her nurse, I don't think she could take it.
Nurse: See how she is when you talk to her. I don't think we can put her off for much longer.
Mr. Davis: I don't need to see how she is. I've lived with her for nearly sixty years. She seems strong but I've always protected her from – well, what I mean is – I love her – I won't have her hurt.

Fig. 7.2 Care plan for Mrs Davis

NAME: Mrs P Davis

HOSPITAL
NO.: 94699

Date	Problem/Deficit	Care to be given	Goal (with date)	Evaluate/Reassess
10.6.85	Risk of pressure sores	Two-hourly turning	Intact skin Review 17.6.85	17.6.85 No pressure sores Continue to monitor
10.6.85	Denial of prognosis	Give her opportunity to discuss future. Pick up cues if she shows desire to discuss future.	That she will have opportunity to accept prognosis. Review 13.6.85.	13.6.85 Patient continues to deny. Re-evaluate 17.6.85 17.6.85 No change
10.6.85	Has poor appetite	Identify preferred foods. Encourage eating but do not insist.	That she will take milky drinks to maintain hydration. Discuss problem with dietician. Review 13.6.85.	13.6.85 Milky drinks taken. Continue to monitor
18.6.85	Mood change? associated with lack of improvement	Allow her to express feelings. Discuss with husband who doesn't want wife told.	That she receives relevant information without husband feeling that his wishes were overridden. Review 20.6.85	20.6.85 Mrs Davis expressing concerns about future and failing spiritual beliefs. Husband expressing feelings of own inability to cope. Agreed nurse should not lie.
20.6.85	Patient concerned for future	Confirm prognosis when she is ready.	That she will accept prognosis in her own time (no date)	21.6.85 Patient's belief about future confirmed. Has asked to go home. Angry, and feels loss of spiritual belief
21.6.85	Failing spiritual belief	Arrange for Minister to visit	Spiritual comfort. Review before discharge	
21.6.85	She wishes to go home	Assess home conditions, support networks, services required, husband's willingness	That she will be able to die at home peacefully	

Nurse (gently): I won't hurt her, and I promise not to raise the subject, but if she asks, I can't lie, can I?

Mr. Davis: Well – Oh, Nurse, how am I going to face it? I can't remember when it wasn't 'us'. She's always put me first, even before the boy – she's everything I have.

In the above exchange, Mr. Davis used the very powerful argument that he knew his wife and therefore knew what was best for her. The nurse, by being gentle but firm, elicited Mr. Davis's fears for a lonely future. His need for assessment and counselling was as great as his wife's. Such fears may be more acute in the elderly since many of their peers and friends may have died and the chances of forming new relationships are reduced.

Some days later, the nurse had a conversation with Mrs. Davis:

Mrs. Davis: I'm sorry about my outburst the other day.

Nurse: Don't apologise. You obviously had a lot on your mind.

Mrs. Davis: I still have – I think I am dying.

Nurse: What makes you say that?

Mrs. Davis: Well, as I said the other day, I'm not getting any better – and George – I know him so well – I know he has something on his mind – and I never have believed that twisted bowel bit – I'm not daft. Yesterday I walked to the toilet but I could barely make it back to bed. I'm tired.

Nurse: You seem to have worked it out, Mrs Davis.

Mrs. Davis (angrily): But I'm not ready. I can't pray anymore, what if there is nothing after this? No God, nothing.

Nurse: I wish I could help. It must be so frightening for you. Would talking to a minister help?

Mrs. Davis: I think he would be shocked – but yes, perhaps – Nurse, how long?

The nurse was unable to give a time to Mrs. Davis but asked her to think of weeks rather than months. She had confirmed Mrs. Davis's suspicions and offered to refer her spiritual problems. Knowing when to refer is a skill which nurses need to develop. This does not mean blocking subjects but, after a patient has aired a concern, listening and assessing and accepting when the problem is one with which she cannot cope alone.

Mrs. Davis cried after she had talked to the nurse and was very quiet for the rest of the day. The minister visited and Mrs. Davis told the nurse that he had seemed to understand how she felt. After her husband had visited that night, Mrs. Davis told Sister that she wished to go home. She had asked George to telephone their daughter-in-law who had offered to come if she was needed.

Evaluation

Faulkner (1985) suggests a number of ways to evaluate care given to patients. Care given to Mrs. Davis was evaluated in terms of whether she had met her potential each day even though that potential was decreasing.

The link between physical health and mental state could be seen when evaluating Mrs. Davis's advance towards acceptance of her prognosis and diagnosis. While she was denying her lack of physical progress, she would force herself to get out of bed, walk to the toilet and sit in the dayroom, even though the nurses did not expect it as they recognised her tiredness. Once acceptance was reached, Mrs. Davis was less hard on herself. She still walked each day but would occasionally ask for a commode, no longer trying to prove anything to herself.

In evaluative terms, Mrs. Davis's acceptance led to more physically comfortable days as only realistic efforts were made. There is often a fear that if a patient knows he is dying, he will 'give up'. This is by no means true. Most people have unfinished business to complete and many are sustained by tasks and ambitions in their final weeks of life.

Also, the preventive care planned for Mrs. Davis had been successful in that the integrity of her skin had been maintained, her mouth and lips were moist and clean and her personal hygiene had been continued by gradually moving from self-care to nursing care. Mobility decreased as did her dietary intake. Her wound had not healed.

If evaluation is measured in terms of physical improvement, then the effectiveness of Mrs. Davis's care would have been rated as a failure except for the preventive aspects, and even here there was a move from self-care to nursing care. By asking if the patient has met her potential each day, a more positive picture emerges.

Mrs. Davis had determined when moves were made in a negative direction. For example, one day she asked if she could have her wash in bed. A few days later she asked if she could have help with washing. The nurses reported this movement from self-care but in terms of evaluation they were satisfied that the patient had reached her potential for self-care on each day.

In terms of mental health, she moved positively towards acceptance without signs of clinical depression, although she did show signs of anger and later, sadness. A positive decision was made by her to spend her final weeks at home.

Discharge

Faulkner (1985) suggests that discharge should be planned well ahead of the expected date. This was not possible for Mrs. Davis since her decision to die at home was unexpected, and her life expectancy was short. However, the information gained from the initial assessment and subsequent conversations with her husband made planning for discharge less complex than it might have been.

Mr. Davis was pleased to be having his wife home but was anxious, especially since his daughter-in-law would not arrive until the day of discharge. Because relationships were good between him and the nursing staff, Mr. Davis was prepared to admit that the house was in a mess and food limited to tins of beans, sardines and chopped meat, a packet of cereal and some potatoes. This honesty led to a home help being arranged so that Mrs. Davis would return to a tidy bungalow with clean sheets on her bed. Meanwhile, the thought of going home had stimulated Mrs. Davis who appeared to enjoy preparing shopping lists and chiding her husband.

Arrangements were also made for the district nurse to visit Mrs. Davis after discharge. Copperman (1983) suggests that 30 percent of the population die at home, cared for by their relatives. This in turn means that there is a need for care and support in the community. In many areas care continues for the family after death in the form of bereavement visiting (Dyne 1981), that is, the district nurse monitors the process of grieving and offers support to the bereaved relatives.

Although Mrs. Davis was dying and was unable to care for herself, her discharge was seen in a positive light. She had had a serious operation, faced a painful reality, accepted a reducing potential and made the positive decision to die at home in her own environment. Much of this was possible because of skilled communication on the part of the nurses. Had her questions been blocked, or false reassurance given, she may have been frustrated, angry and unable to decide what to do. As a result she may have died in hospital, a victim of collusion.

Physically, skilled nursing care aided a comfortable return home. Had pressure sores or a mouth infection developed, relatives may have had difficulty in giving adequate care, even with the help of a district nurse. Although goals for improvement had not been set, Mrs. Davis had been given high levels of physical and psychological care which allowed her to die with dignity.

Some weeks later, Mr. Davis visited the ward to say that his wife had died peacefully after spending her last weeks organising the household so that her husband could manage to survive alone after her death. He said that although there had been sad and serious times together, there had been a lot of love and laughter, especially when he had attempted to make gravy under his daughter-in-law's watchful eye. He was sad but felt that his wife had had 'a good life'.

Dying and the Deficit model

If the patients' needs, derived from deficits, are to be met, it is essential that care is planned in the light of the patients' perceptions of and reactions to their current state. Nowhere is this more true than in the care of the terminally ill patient since no assumptions can be made of what dying means to any one individual.

Because each individual is unique, the deficits arising from a terminal illness will be many and varied, especially psychological deficits. Physical deficits are only different from those of patients who will live in that recovery is not possible. In all aspects except for evaluation, high levels of nursing care are mandatory no matter what the prognosis.

The nursing process, focused on deficits perceived by patients, allows for individual assessment of each terminally ill patient. Such an approach should enhance the care of the elderly dying patient in that each person's dying will be an individual event rather than a 'normal' expectation of old age. Of course dying is inevitable for everyone but there is seldom a 'good' time to die. There is always something else to be achieved and a future to be believed in. The elderly are perhaps more aware of their mortality as they see partners, friends and peers die but even this cannot be assumed. Mr. Davis at 80 was sad and lonely after his wife's death but did not think of dying. Some months after the funeral he started to take a widow of 70 years to whist drives and began to talk of a future again.

Other elderly people may react differently. The death of a partner may cause the survivor to 'give up' and die within a short time. Assessment of each patient should elicit attitudes to life and reactions to deficits in relationships and to dying itself.

Models for nursing

There is an increasing interest in models for nursing. Many overlap in their concepts. For example, Roper's model (1980) is based on activities of daily living, while Orem (1971) bases her model on self-care. Implicit in these is the concept of need and, therefore, deficit. The deficit model, because it is based on an individual's perception of his world, also incorporates the concepts of daily living activities and self-care, but is more concerned with the patient's reactions to deficits caused by illness. The thread that links these models is that of nursing being a dynamic process. In the care of the elderly dying patient and his family, this allows for creative care for each patient rather than routine nursing of a 'Cinderella' section of society.

The notion of helping a patient to reach his potential is seen to be crucial in evaluating care for the elderly dying patient, and in this respect the deficit model which allows for goals to move in a negative direction is seen to be particularly useful. A potential weakness is that there may be problems for the patient who is at the stage of denial, since rationalisations will be needed to explain a worsening condition.

It can be argued that, providing the nurse understands the patient's perception of his state, progress can be made towards acceptance when the patient gives cues that he is ready to do so. In Mrs. Davis's case, the nurse, by appreciating that there was an underlying cause for anger and aggression on the part of the patient, was able to assess and deal with the psychological problems presented. In this instance, using a model in which it is accepted that goals can be set in a negative direction was successful in that the patient died with dignity in the place of her choosing with the full co-operation of her relatives.

Finally, the deficit model, by including all aspects of an individual's life, can lead nursing to give due attention to the patient's family. They too have deficits and needs which are caused by, or related to, the patient and his current illness. In terminal care, relatives face a future which is bound to change. Nurses can support individuals as they try to accept and cope with that change.

References

Brewin TB 1977 The cancer patient: communication and morale. *British Medical Journal*, 2: 1623–1627.

Brink TL 1979 *Geriatric psychotherapy*. Human Sciences Press, New York.

Cooper DL 1983 *Stress research. Issues for the eighties*. Wiley, Chichester.

Copperman H 1983 *Dying at home.* HM&M, Aylesbury.

Dyne B (Ed) 1981 *Bereavement visiting.* King Edward's Hospital Fund for London, London.

Faulkner A 1985 *Nursing—a creative approach.* Bailliere Tindall, London.

Gingell J 1985 Nursing practice and accountability. In: Sykes, M. (Ed) *Licensed to practise.* Bailliere Tindall, London.

Henderson V 1960 *Basic principles of nursing care.* International Council of Nurses, London.

Kubler-Ross E 1973 *On death and dying.* Tavistock, London.

Kubler-Ross E 1975 *Death, the final stage of growth.* Prentice Hall, New York.

Mackintosh J 1977 *Communication and awareness in a cancer ward.* Croom Helm, London.

McFarlane J & Castledine G 1982 *A guide to the practice of nursing using the nursing process.* Mosby, London.

Maslow AH 1954 *Motivation and personality.* 2nd Ed. Harper & Row, New York.

Norton D, McLaren R & Exton-Smith A 1962 reissued 1975. *Investigations of geriatric nursing problems in hospital.* Churchill Livingstone, Edinburgh.

Orem DE 1971 *Nursing: concepts of practice.* McGraw Hill, New York.

Parsons T 1966 On becoming a patient. In: Folter, K. & Deck, E. (Eds) *A sociological framework for patient care.* Wiley, New York.

Rogers CR 1961 *On becoming a person.* Houghton Mifflin, Boston.

Roper N, Logan WW & Tierney AJ 1980 *The elements of nursing.* Churchill Livingstone, Edinburgh.

Simpson MA 1975 Teaching about death and dying. In: Raven, R. S. (Ed) *The dying patient.* Pitman Medical, London.

Tait A *et al.* 1982 Improving communication skills. *Nursing Times*, 78, 51: 2181–2184.

Index